Closets are for Clothes

RICHARD HARRIS

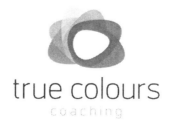

true colours
coaching

First paperback edition printed 2010 in the United Kingdom

Published by True Colours Coaching LLP

http://www.truecolourscoaching.com

http://www.closetsareforclothes.co.uk

British Library Cataloguing in Publication Data
A catalogue record for this book is available from the British Library

ISBN: 978-0-9565579-0-2

Cover designed by IANAR - **www.ianar.deviantart.com**

Printed in Great Britain by Lightning Source

Closets

are for

Clothes

UNDERSTANDING AND
CELEBRATING EVERYTHING GAY!

LIVING A HAPPY AND SUCCESSFUL
LIFE OUTSIDE THE CLOSET

WWW.CLOSETSAREFORCLOTHES.CO.UK

For Andrew, who has and always will be a constant support and my rock. Forever a better version of me, I thank my lucky stars everyday that I found you. You are the greatest person I have ever met.

For Mam and Dad who never turned their back on me when the world so often did. Your love and support is the reason I am where I am today. You gave me life, you fought to make it a happy one and I love you more than life itself.

For Julian, Claire and William. My thanks to both of you for being there, also for our special Nephew whose intelligent wit and kind nature will allow him to be anything he wants to be – he's the most treasured gift that we have ever been given.

For Nanny Beatrice, it was you who taught me so much about life at such a young age. You were my best friend and now my Guardian Angel. I love you. And for my Grampy Tom, Nanny and Grampy Harris whom I only know through the wonderful memories you gave Mam and Dad. Thank you for doing such a great job with them.

For Auntie Joyce, one of life's biggest characters, you would always take my side even when I was wrong, yet put me gently but firmly in my place. I can't count the times I think about you in a single day, I'll miss you everyday for the rest of my life. And for Uncle Doug, a wonderful man, I'm so proud to call you Uncle. You were the wind beneath Auntie Joyce's wings, your love and support of the family makes us infinitely richer for having you.

For my Aunties, thank you for the joy you have brought to my life; and Auntie Beat for always going along with the joke when I stole your ornaments, or for never looking at me silly when I used to wear your stilettos (though I was only four or five).

For my wonderful cousins – there are just too many to mention.

For Cheryl and Martin, thank you for allowing me to join your family and to share my life with your wonderful son.

Acknowledgements

Closets Are For Clothes would not have been possible without the continued support of my friend and Editor, Hazel Bagley. She went above and beyond in both of the aforementioned roles and it was her sensitive direction (and a whole heap of laughter) that made this whole experience an enjoyable one.

I would to thank Lorraine Bevan for her remarkable proof reading skills.

My thanks and appreciation goes to the wonderful people below (in alphabetical order to save arguments). These people have made my life far more enriched for being a part of it at sometime or another.

Andrew Bloom ▪ Angela Sheehy ▪ Angelina Algieri ▪ Auntie Beatrice & Uncle Huw ▪ Auntie Doreen & Uncle Herb ▪ Auntie Gwen & Uncle Harold ▪ Auntie Janice & Uncle Mal ▪ Auntie Lou ▪ Auntie Marion & Uncle Ron ▪ Barbara Harries ▪ Barry Cheeseman ▪ Bridgette & Alan Burnett ▪ Chris Davies ▪ Christine & Mike Merritt ▪ Claire 'Patricia' Barrett ▪ Corinne Jones ▪ Curly Martin ▪ Dave Griffiths ▪ Dave, Hilary & Bethan Williams ▪ Denzil Hopkins ▪ Emma Williams ▪ Eve, Geraint, Emie, Rohan & Harry Jenkins ▪ Geraint Williams & Family ▪ Gloria & Bryan Pegler & Aunt Sal ▪ Greg Miller ▪ Hannah Davies ▪ Jane Stone ▪ Jay Harley ▪ Jennifer Abell ▪ Joyce Piper ▪ Karen Newton ▪ Kate Thomas ▪ Kelly Flay & The Bread Babes ▪ Laila Quattrini ▪ Laura Skidmore ▪ Laura Thain ▪ Lisa Geraci ▪ Lisa Pritchard ▪ Liz Lamprey ▪ Lorraine, Geoff & Family ▪ Lowri Oliver ▪ Lynda & Graham Eddolls ▪ Lynda Edwards ▪ Lynne Jones ▪ Lynsey Williams ▪ Maxine Richards ▪ Menna & Sian Cook ▪ Mildred Eddolls ▪ Morgan Lloyd ▪ Nicola Thornton ▪ Rachel Lambert ▪ Rhiannon & Dave Anthony ▪ Ria Darch ▪ Richard & Lisa Crowther ▪ Sally Jones ▪ Stephen Price ▪ Steven James ▪ Suzanne Evans ▪ Teri Knight, Granny Smith, Claire Pullen, Sarah Davies & Beth Norman ▪ Tim Hodges ▪ Uncle Robert & Auntie Mandy ▪ Vanessa Wilkinson-Hughes ▪ Wendy 'Chardonnay' Owen ▪ The Zodiac Musketeers – Carrie, Denise, Diane, Gareth, Gerry, Karen, Ruth & Vicky

Contents

Introduction

You have decided to purchase this book for a reason.

You know what it is like to be stuffed right at the back of the closet with very little room to move with all those clothes, shoes and not to mention the skeletons. It can be a dark and lonely place especially when you do not have a flashlight. I have written this book in a "no-holds-barred" fashion in order to look at the accomplishments and complications that are part and parcel of life when you realise that you are different from the rest of the people in your world. As you first begin to look at yourself as gay, lesbian or bi-sexual it leaves you with feelings of dread, you know you are different and with this comes the emotional rollercoaster ride, just because you are attracted to those who are the same sex.

It is natural to think that this automatically removes you from the world leaving you locked in a closet where you experience life through the crack between the doors but it needn't. Think of how great life can be when you decide to open up and tell those whom you love about the real you, and when they accept you for whom you are. You are not alone, there are millions who understand your situation, there are those who have broken free of the closet and there are those who remain locked inside. Allow this book to be your flashlight so that you see the clearer picture that will have you grabbing for the handle so you can set yourself free. You will discover the real person that is hiding inside that closet, a person that is a true individual worthy of love, respect and acceptance for being gay, lesbian or bi-sexual. These are just labels by the way; they in no way define who you are as a person.

You are not alone, there are millions of people who are gay, lesbian and bi-sexual who understand the uphill struggle of coming to terms with knowing that deep down you are different from everyone else. This handbook has been created with due care and attention to educate and act as a helping hand for you, friends, parents and members of your family who will need to adjust to the new (and improved) you.

CHAPTER ONE

Catching The Right Bus And Batting For The Right Side – What Is It All About?

I want to congratulate you for choosing this book, as you read through you will realise that you are not the only person who feels different from the rest of the world because you are attracted to people of the same sex. When we begin school very quickly we learn to act 'normal', we want to fit in, we want to be accepted. What is 'normal' anyway? Well, my interpretation of normal is I wake up each morning feeling happy, comfortable in the skin I am in. I treat people with the respect they deserve and I give thanks to be alive. That is it for me.

This is not the case for everyone; there are those who are so misunderstood by others for the way they feel they wish that life would just end. However, there is a lot of life to live. Being gay is only a small part of who a person is, there is so much more besides.

This book started out a lot smaller than I anticipated. It was written based on my own experiences, but then I opened it up to the world. I asked individuals from all over the globe, from all walks of life to share their experiences. Many of them feature in this book as 'case studies'. Remember, these 'case studies' are real people, with blood running through their veins and each has feelings and a story to tell.

Tim's Story

"I remember showing signs of homosexuality when I was four years old. However, I only realised that the feelings I had meant I was gay at around eleven years old, I am fourteen now.

I live in South East Asia; I attend a Christian High School which is very strict against homosexuality. I often, no, ALWAYS get offended when we have topics in Science about homosexuality and people laugh and make fun of it. I feel they are laughing at me and people who are like me. Now at the age of fourteen I can appreciate that life is tough.

I am very scared to come out. In fact, I'm really afraid that someone I know might see this book and find out it is me. I tried coming out a while ago; I decided to do a trial run on a friend so I told him I was bi-sexual. He was a really awesome friend before I said anything, now he doesn't talk to me.

After telling my friend I was bi-sexual (which I'm not, I'm gay), I was anticipating that he would be gay too and understand what I was going through. I had to face facts, he wasn't. Things went horribly wrong for me, I felt really terrible.

I am scared though.

I am suffering an internal battle because my religion and culture does not understand my feelings. I'd explode with tears if everyone didn't accept me for who I really am. I have contemplated suicide at least four times in my lifetime. I overcame them by thinking about something that was worth living for".

Which Bus To Catch? The Gay Bus, The Straight Bus Or The Bi Bus?

We live in a world that takes great comfort in neatly labelling and packaging everything, which social group we belong to, which area we live in and where we were born. A person's sexuality does not escape the wrath of being labelled.

We will start this at the very beginning because according to Julie Andrews this is a very good place to start, and what Julie says goes. Well it does if you are a gay man.

People who are attracted to the same sex, like you, me and millions of other people are known as *gay*, this is a popular term or more formally *homosexual*. Those who are attracted to the opposite sex are called *straight* or *heterosexual*. The term gay covers both genders but it is usually associated with men, females who are attracted to other females are usually known as *lesbian*. In addition there are many people who are sexually attracted to both sexes these are *bi-sexual*.

If you have never thought of yourself as special for being gay, then just remember you are. Gay people have been the subject of name calling long before it was thrust into the public eye and being gay became fashionable. Gay men have, at one time in their life, been called fags, poofs, queers, homos, faggots, shirt-lifters, shit shovellers, arse bandits and benders. I am sure there are other equally side-splitting names that I have forgotten to mention.

The one I dislike most is the word faggot. I looked it up after a friend of mine asked how it derived, this is what I found: The word faggot is a term of measurement for a bundle of sticks and straw which were used during the 1600s to help fuel the burning of witches at the stake. Others who also suffered the same fate were gay people, but before being burnt they were forced to collect bundles of sticks with which they would be burnt. When the bundles of sticks had come to an end, the gay people were thrown on to keep the fire burning for the witches.

Gay females have also been called dykes, lesbos, lezzers and rug munchers.

The bi-sexual men and women are usually just called greedy!

These labels are hurtful and spiteful and do nothing but destroy a person's self-worth. I know reading these slurs may bring back hurtful echoes of what those small minded individuals once said to you. Sticks and stones... yeah right. Who ever coined that phrase was never subject to being regularly disparaged by vile euphemisms about an aspect of themselves they never chose or couldn't change.

Even today an individual's sexuality or sexual orientation, whatever you call it is still a hot topic, people like nothing more than pocketing people into what they believe to be true. Sexuality can be a broad term as it will cover those who are homosexual, heterosexual or bi-sexual.

However, there is more to being gay, straight or bi than who people are attracted to. These labels don't always fit with a person. We are individuals; we are talking about people's feelings, not just about who they share their lives with. There is absolutely no need to live up to a stereotype or label. The most important thing is to discover who you are and feel comfortable. Once you have mastered this, only then will people understand the real you and love you because you love yourself.

A person's sexuality is a little more complex than black is black and white is white. I have met a broad spectrum of people who have had same sex relationships in the past, in school or university but then go on to settle down in a heterosexual relationship and never looked back.

You are a gift; your sexuality is only a small part of who you are, although at times it seems to be a huge issue for you and some others too. I suspect that the people who really matter will care more for you being a good, decent human being. Others will be drawn to someone who is honest, kind, considerate and respectable, irrespective of their sexuality.

Why Am I Batting For This Side?

Unfortunately life is not a game of baseball, we don't line up in front of the team captains and hope to be selected to play on our desired team, it is determined way before we take our first breath.

Once you have realised that you are gay, you will have grown up asking 'Why am I gay?' it is expected, I did too. This is the million pound question; it is right up there with 'What is the meaning of life'. By the way I have the answer to both questions, but we will stick to the matter in hand for the time being. I spent a lot of my time whilst growing up with other questions whirling around in my head such as, 'Why me, and not them?' and 'How can I change this?' I just wanted to be like all the other boys and girls in my class. I found myself trapped in a world where they can put a man on the moon, clone sheep, reproduce human organs on the back of mice, allow people to sail and fly safely around the world nonetheless they could not change my feelings towards those of the same sex. Though there are many theories and many studies have been undertaken, no-one fully understands or has definite proof of what determines or influences our sexuality. I am not a man of science therefore I have no fact but I can hypothesise: I believe that homosexuality and bi-sexuality is genetic. I strongly believe, as do many others that we are born with our sexuality. It has been claimed that our sexuality is influenced after we are born and it forms itself based on childhood events and the environment we are brought up in. This theory is quashed by twins who are raised identically and share the same life experiences, but only one is gay.

There are many theories that have been reached in order to pinpoint why a person is born other than heterosexual. Some say that a child's sexuality is determined if they have a strong female influence, primarily the mother, and an absent or disinterested father. Another theory is that there are tell tale signs of the child's sexual orientation by what toys/type of play the child seems to be drawn to. I have encountered many mums who have dissuaded their sons from playing with dolls based on this notion. This has not been scientifically confirmed, playing with dolls or being a sensitive boy is unlikely to determine your little boy's future sexual tendencies. Likewise, little girls who climb trees or want a train set; this does not influence their sexuality.

Generally, I find people are afraid of that which they do not understand from their personal experience. Those people believe that to be gay is an unnatural digression from what is deemed 'normal'. In today's world there is no 'normal' any more, everyone is a unique individual. There is much confusion about what makes a person *want* to be gay. In fact you don't *want* to be anything; you just *are* and have to deal with it (which is where this book comes in!) You just want to be like your friends, siblings and those that pass you by in the street. These people didn't choose to be straight in the same way you didn't choose to be gay, you must accept that you are 'normal' and it is natural to have feelings towards the sex you are attracted to. Though the feelings of abnormality and isolation are understandable you have to embrace the special person you are and love the life you have and the fantastic future you have ahead.

What's Wrong With Being Gay?

In a word: Nothing. Disliking the feeling of being different is natural and being gay doesn't mean you are in the wrong or by any means inferior to those who are heterosexual. Indeed there are many who think it is a choice, but I can assure you that no-one chooses to be gay.

It has been mentioned before and I will mention it again, 'People are afraid of what they don't understand'. *Homophobia*, and no this not a fear of water, this is a prejudice or dislike of homosexuals through ignorance. More often than not it derives from the lack of understanding of homosexuality and bi-sexuality (remember we just talked about this). Unfortunately, those with homophobic beliefs only learn to change their perception when it immediately affects them and even then they may chose not to learn and continue to be small minded. As you make your journey through life you will encounter a lot of people who are comfortable with homosexuality. It has become more widely understood and accepted since there have been more iconic figures in the public domain speaking about their homosexuality. The repeal of 'Section 28' as a result of many marches has pushed it into the political arena.

Do Something About It

You can make a huge difference right now. This exercise can change your outlook of the world and those you inhabit it with, more importantly it will change the outlook of yourself. Get a pen and paper; write down the one thing that you feel most uncomfortable about.

For example, 'I'm unhappy being gay'

It doesn't have to be that, it can be anything that might be running around your head now. The things that are coming to mind are hurtful and painful and it is these beliefs that are holding you back from being happy with yourself. Write down as many as you can think of and then put your pen down. Take a breath.

Done it? If you haven't done it then try it! What have you got to lose?

Done it now?

Right you are starting to bug me now. You picked this book up for a reason, and that reason was to understand that being gay is not a negative state; it is a natural part of who you are. Get that pen and paper, there is very little effort required and this will only make you happier, it can't make you feel worse so there has to be some good in it.

Right, now that you have done that, well done for doing it, the more you practice what I am showing you, you will notice a significant difference to the way you feel about yourself and others.

Take those thoughts you have noted down and write the opposite in positive terms.

For example, where you have put, "I'm unhappy being gay", write "I am comfortable and happy with being gay" (or whatever else you wrote)

You can also write variations of this statement such as:-

"I love myself and therefore I love and accept myself for being gay" (or whatever else you wrote)

Remember, it is *your* statement so write it how you feel comfortable. You might want to write one for each of the issues you noted down.

Once you have written them, either copy them onto a card in your best handwriting or print them off the computer and stick it around your environment where you will see it on a regular basis e.g. kitchen cupboards, bathroom mirror, noticeboard - you get the idea! I promise that it does work.

If you can't pin it up at home in case someone might see it, write it in your journal and look at it when you are at your lowest, at your happiest or just whenever you want. You will not believe them at first, of course not, you have grown up being told otherwise. These things you have written in the positive tense are your new truth; you just need to believe them for them to be true.

Remember, if you know any straight people who might benefit from this exercise then tell them about it. It's not exclusive to us gays you know.

There is something that is very important to remember and I mention it now as it is the underlying theme of the entire book and that is: Being gay is only a small part of who you are. You will have many titles in life, as a male you will be a son, perhaps brother, uncle, best friend, boyfriend, and partner. As a female you will be a daughter perhaps sister, auntie, best friend, girlfriend, and partner. There is more to you than being labelled as gay and it is important to hear this message early on through life.

PATRICK HARRISON'S STORY

"I am fifteen years of age now; I was around thirteen when I first started noticing that I was attracted to guys. It is difficult because I am only now coming to terms with my sexuality and I am being bullied at school for being gay yet I have told no-one, people call me names and bug me about it. I know what I am and they know what I am but the more they bug me the more I want to hide it. I have recently come out to my mom, she is having a hard time accepting it but is trying to be supportive, I have told some close friends and they have taken it very well.

Telling those few people has allowed me to feel better about myself and I can actually be myself around them. I just wish it didn't hurt my mom so much, I can understand why she is hurting but this is all beyond my control. Coming out to the few I have mentioned is the best thing I have ever done, it was probably the hardest but it does pay off in the end.

I live in Virginia in the US and was raised to be a devout Catholic but the message I get from those who attend church is they are against me and
8

those like me. It's a shame, I thought religion was about love, forgiveness, accepting others and not judging. I stand corrected.

I wish people would understand how I feel and I am glad that this book has been written because I am hoping it will help inform my mom and any other friends or family members that might have difficulty understanding what it is like to be born different without having the choice in the first place".

CHAPTER TWO

A History Of Homosexuality Since Time Began

This chapter will give you a brief overview of the gay movement over the centuries and as we all love gossip columns and magazines there is mention of many of the people who were gay, lesbian or bi-sexual, those who helped enforce it and those who abolished it.

I have always loved history; it was a subject that my mother encouraged me to pursue from a very young age. It's a real shame that when I reached Comprehensive School my History teacher took an instant dislike to me. I remember my first lesson with him, he said "Harris? Harris? Do you have a brother that has just left this school?" I replied "Yes, sir". His face dropped and from that moment on he had no time for me. No matter what I did, it was never right.

My favourite subject matter was, and still is the British monarchy, the Tudor dynasty, Queen Victoria and those who pre-dated 1936. I grew up with the classic films that depicted Tudor life, *Anne of a Thousand Days* with Welsh iconic legend Richard Burton; and *Mary, Queen of Scots* and *Elizabeth R* with Glenda Jackson. One day he gave us an assignment to write about Queen Elizabeth I and the Spanish Armada, I raced home and though I would stray from the piddling fact sheet he gave me and wrote a wonderful piece giving great detail of the event, I used real facts from the books my mother has collected over the years and some that she had bought for me. I translated everything into the Welsh language; attending a Welsh school meant that all lessons were delivered in Welsh. He didn't even bother marking it, I stood in front of his desk as he skimmed through it, reciting a catalogue of facts that I had mentioned that he didn't even want to know. This is disheartening for a boy of twelve, as he could obviously see I had a keen interest but he doused any passion I had for his lesson there and then. After that I occasionally spent lessons in the hallway having been sent out of class for lack of interest, I had as much interest in his lessons as he had in me.

I hope you find this informative, there might be a lot of information in parts but sit back and enjoy it. We have come a long way to where we are now, we should appreciate and embrace the freedom we have now been given. The view of same sex relationships has changed greatly over the years – indeed since the beginning of time. We have moved from same sex relationships being socially acceptable and proper, to being seen as a sin, disallowed with severe punishment and the death penalty.

B.C.

In Greece around 400BC, marriage between two men is not legally recognised, although long-term relationships and partnerships do go on. These partnerships between men are similar to the heterosexual relationships of the day, however there is about a generation gap in age between them and this is called pederasty. The elder partner is seen as a mentor and the younger partner being in their adolescent years, between thirteen and twenty years of age, will learn from their mentor. A period of courtship goes on; the young male who gives in too quickly is seen as someone who has easy virtues, and those who hold out too long gain the reputation as a seducer who have no intentions of fulfilling their expectation.

One member of each of these relationships assumes a passive sexual role and the other, an active role (penetrator). It is the elder in the relationship, or the mentor, who is the active partner as it's seen as a display of masculinity, adulthood and high social status. The passive role belongs to the younger partner as it is associated with femininity, youth and the lower orders. Homosexuality is accepted but transvestism and effeminate men are not, they are mocked and ridiculed. It is thought that homosexuality between men; especially fighting men in the army boosts the fighting spirit.

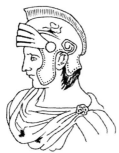

Alexander The Great

Alexander III of Macedon also known as Alexander the Great has the vision to conquer the entire world. He conquers the Persian Empire and extends his rule over Greece to as far as India. Alexander is romantically involved with his childhood best friend, Hephaestion. Both men are beautiful beyond compare; they grow up together and fight side by side as they begin their conquest. When Persia is under Alexander's rule, Alexander takes three wives, but his love for Hephaestion is infinite. Alexander also takes another male lover, a Persian subject, which causes upset not because he is male, but a Persian. It was hoped that Alexander would take a Macedonian or Greek bride but all three wives were foreign to his homeland and considered barbarians. When Hephaestion dies Alexander knows that he will be reunited with his lover at the point of his death.

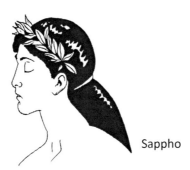

Sappho

Relationships between female homosexuals are not overly discussed or documented, of course it is still present even if not documented, and there is still prejudice. It is alleged that Sappho, the female poet from Lesbos is attracted to women. Sappho is born around 630BC in Lesbos (which name has generated the word *lesbian*, linking the historical figure of Sappho to the whole of female homosexuality. As demonstrated by the use of the word *sapphic* as another synonymous of sexual relationships between women).

Homosexuality in ancient Rome around the period of 200BC sees a period that is both of condemnation and social acceptance. Bi-sexuality is common during this time, among men certainly, although there are those who have relationships exclusively with men and who identify as homosexual.

Lex Scantinia is introduced around 149BC; this is an ancient Roman law brought in during the Roman Republic that rules sexual behaviour resulting in death for those who take part in same sex relationships. This law is only for free-born men, slaves are excluded from this. Free-born men can do whatever they wish with slaves as long as it does not contravene the law. There are those who engage in sexual acts with slaves, however this is seen as a means of punishment for misbehaviour or disobedience – which to me is tantamount to rape.

Let's take a quick journey through time and note significant events throughout history as well as some famous names that you might not have known were gay, lesbian or bi-sexual.

Before we go back and visit those events and meet the infamous people that created them, it is important to remember that being gay is not a 'new thing'. The Roman Empire saw many of its Emperors support and indeed take part in same sex relationships. Nero and Elagabalus both of them Roman Emperors went on to marry men whilst other Emperors had gay lovers as well as wives. In around 80BC it is said that Julius Caesar has a love affair with the King of Bithynia. Transvestism and effemininity are not accepted, and any free-born or high ranking inhabitant found performing oral sex or playing the role of the passive partner will be publically disgraced.

1st Century

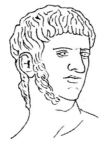

Emperor Nero

Nero becomes Emperor of the Roman Empire in the year 54 and marries a man by the name of Pythagoras; Nero is the "wife" during this first marriage. When it comes to an end, Nero then moves his attention to another man and this time becomes the "husband" within the same sex marriage to Sporus, whom Nero has had castrated. The relationship between man and Emperor continues over time as Trajan, one of the most popular of Roman Emperors who rules in the year 97, notoriously has an eye for young men.

2nd Century

Roman Emperor, Hadrian who has ruled since 117 has a male lover too, Antinous who is Greek. Their love affair ends tragically when they are both on a tour of Egypt, an accident occurs whilst travelling on the barge resulting in Antinous being thrown into the Nile. Antinous dies and Hadrian lives out the rest of his days a shattered man glorifying Antinous' name, it is said that the death of his partner has driven him close to insanity. Hadrian dies in the year 138.

3rd Century

The year 218 sees the reign of the Roman Emperor, Elagabalus, who marries five women during a short succession and then marries Zoticus, a young man of impeccable dimensions – he is an athlete. They have a very lavish public ceremony with full support of the public. It is said that Elagabalus has transgender issues as he wears large amounts of make-up and it is rumoured that he offered a substantial sum of money to his physician in return for giving him female genitalia. Elagabalus and his mother are both brutally murdered and their bodies cast aside with no pomp or ceremony.

There was a change in attitude between the years 244 and 249, the Roman Emperor Philippus I attempts and fails to outlaw homosexual prostitution which has been widely accepted in Rome, so much so it has been taxed and considered suitable.

4th Century

It is during the year 342 that the first law in opposition of same sex marriage is brought in by Roman Emperors Constantine II, Constantius II and Constans, who are three brothers who rule jointly over the Empire since the death of their father, Constantine I. The year 390 sees the Emperors Theodosius I, Valentinian II and Arcadius proclaim that any same sex relationships or homosexual sex is to be seen as sin against God and illegal. The penalty for those charged under this law is public execution by burning.

5th Century

The year 476 sees the end of the Roman Empire as it is known, and with it ends the many tales about homosexuality within the Roman Empire. It is clear to see how "When in Rome, do as the Romans do" seems more appealing, or at least it was back then.

Time passes and things go very quiet as we travel through time, of course there are still men and women who participate in same sex relationships, and there are still changes in peoples tolerance of same sex relationships, at some times customary, and at others unacceptable.

(The Roman Emperors were not the only royals who were identified as gay, lesbian and bi-sexual. It would seem that there was an epidemic of British royalty who also appreciated the beauty of the same sex – keep reading).

11th Century

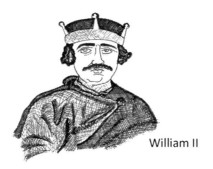

William II

It is the 11th Century, and William II is the second monarch to rule England. William is the son of the first British monarch, William I who is known as William the Conqueror. William II is open about his homosexuality; he is an arrogant man who quarrels frequently with the Church and extorts money from his subjects. In 1100 he is found dead in the New Forest, he has been killed by a single arrow. There are many reports as to how this happens, some say accidental death from a stray arrow, and others believe murder. His brother Henry I who succeeds him is also accused – is he homophobic perhaps? Nevertheless, those who are with William flee and leave him in fear of being convicted of his death.

12th Century

The beginning of a new century, and the Council of London announces most vehemently that homosexuality is a sinful act.

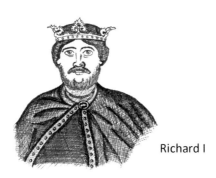

Richard I

Richard I who is known as the mighty Richard the Lionheart is ruler of Great Britain. He becomes king in 1189 and it is said that he involves himself with other men at court and it is documented that on one occasion Richard shares a bed with King Philip II of France as a symbol of unity between the two countries – that's their story and they are sticking to it.

13th Century

Thomas Aquinas, an Italian priest of the Roman Catholic Church states publicly that homosexual acts are deemed second only to murder in the eyes of God. In 1283 the French law commands that homosexuals are not only put to death by burning but that all their properties are forfeited also.

14th Century

Meanwhile back in England...

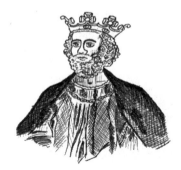

Edward II

King Edward II of England rules Great Britain, he ascends the throne in 1307 as he succeeds his father Edward I. Edward II is infatuated with Piers Gaveston whom he dubs the Earl of Cornwall. In 1312 Thomas Plantagenet, Earl of Lancaster and cousin to the king summons his own private army to separate Gaveston from the king, they both run to Scarborough where Edward leaves him so that he can raise his own army against the Earl. Gaveston is captured and taken to Warwickshire and he is slain by the Earl of Lancaster's swordsmen and then beheaded as he lay dying. Edward avenges his lover's death ten years later when he executes his cousin in 1322. Five years pass and Edward dies a most vicious death, as his wife Isabella over-throws him and has him imprisoned at Berkeley Castle. One evening Edward is dragged from his bed, by Isabella's men, and he is suffocated. That's not all, during the suffocation; a tube is inserted into his back passage to allow a red-hot plumber's iron to be pushed inside in order to burn all major organs. This is perhaps favourable as there are no visible causes of death should his body be examined – talk about a "hot rod".

Edward and Isabella's son, Edward III is pronounced king.

Throughout Europe gay men are being burned for their homosexuality. France introduces a punishment that first offenders found performing same sex activity will have a testicle removed, the second offence results in the removal of the penis and the third is death. Females who take part in same sex activities will be mutilated and put to death. It's great to see that for women that there is no warning system. It's death at first strike. It's definitely a case of don't do as I do, but do as I say.

Meanwhile back in England...

Some time has passed and Edward III dies in 1377 leaving the crown to his son, Richard II, he is ten years old. Whispers at court say that Richard is homosexual; he has a very close relationship with Robert de Vere, Earl of Oxford. Robert dies in France in 1395 from the wounds he obtains after an attack from a wild boar. Richard II has his embalmed body brought back to Great Britain; Richard wishes to see his friend one last time and kisses his hand. The close relationship between the two causes much commotion and the funeral is snubbed by some of King Richard's court. Richard is over-thrown in 1399 and then dies a year later at the hands of his cousin who becomes the next to rule, Henry IV.

15th Century

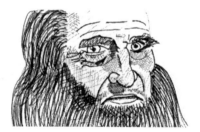

Leonardo Da Vinci

The same old things are going on around world, and Leonardo Da Vinci creator of such masterpieces as The Last Supper and the Mona Lisa is charged in a court of law in Florentine for homosexual relations with three other men, all three however are released and found not guilty.

16th Century

1532 sees the Holy Roman Empire declare that homosexuality is punishable by death as it is a sin against God and the Holy Church. The following year King Henry VIII, who needs absolutely no introduction passes the Buggery Act 1533 and pronounces that all same sex activity will result in death. Then twenty years later in 1553, Mary I, daughter of Henry VIII and his first wife Catherine of Aragon, comes to the throne and reverses the religious changes that Henry VIII had put into action. Mary also removes all of the laws passed by Henry VIII even the Buggery Act. Following Mary's death in 1558, Elizabeth I, daughter of Henry VIII and Anne Boleyn ascends the throne and reinstates the Buggery Act along with all other laws that apply to same sex behaviour. It is all fun and games during the Tudor dynasty.

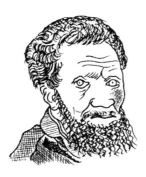

Michelangelo

A notable figure that is suspected of being homosexual is the Italian painter, sculpture and architect, Michelangelo. He has a catalogue of famous works to his name, namely his statue of David which he completes in 1504. He comes under scrutiny about his sexuality because of the company he keeps and his erotic creations. The question is, can a genius that creates a 17 foot marble statue of an Adonis by the name of David, really be straight?

17th Century

The 17th Century continues to witness countries from all parts of the globe condemning homosexuality and persecuting all those who take part in same sex relationships. This is being fuelled by the strength of the Catholic Church. What is perceived as unnatural by those who don't understand, is completely natural to those attracted by the same sex.

Let's go now to England and have a little look what's happening there...

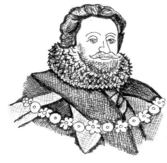

James I (VI of Scotland)

King James I of England first becomes King James VI of Scotland in 1567 when he is one year old, then later takes the English throne following the death of Elizabeth I in 1603. James' mother, Mary, Queen of Scots was imprisoned and put to death by James' predecessor (and Godmother) Elizabeth I. When James is thirteen years old he falls in love with his male cousin, Esme Stewart who is thirty-seven. The young king elevates Esme Stewart to the Duke of Lennox. In 1582 at the age of sixteen, James is lured to Ruthven Castle as a guest; however he is held prisoner by Scottish nobles and will only be released when he renounces his lover and banishes him out of Scotland. James is held for ten months and in order to secure his release he agrees to banish the Duke of Lennox. The Duke flees to France and dies soon after. James shows very little interest in women throughout his life and is commended for his chastity in his youth, yet when he reaches the age of twenty-three he marries the fourteen year old Anne of Denmark.

The year 1606, after three years on the English throne, James falls for Robert Carr who is intelligent as well as beautiful. Carr is given the Earldom of Somerset and there is much unhappiness at court about Carr's popularity, so those who oppose Robert Carr attempt to turn James' favour to another man, George Villiers. James being as predictable as ever welcomes Villiers as a lover and he makes him Baron Whaddon, Viscount Villiers and Earl of Buckingham in very quick succession. James not feeling that he had decorated him enough then elevates him to Marquess of Buckingham, Earl of Coventry and finally the Duke of Buckingham – he is the most decorated subject outside of the royal family and over time will gain the reputation as the most decorated subject in all history. James' reign ends in 1625 with the Duke of Buckingham at his side. It is James' reign that saw the capture of the masterminds behind the Gunpowder Plot of 1605.

Time passes and England sees the reign of Charles I who is beheaded by Oliver Cromwell who is made Lord Protector and England is turned into a Republican Commonwealth. Then Charles II, son of Charles I and grandson of James I is restored as rightful monarch and assumes the throne in 1660, two years after Cromwell's death. Charles II dies after a glorious reign and his brother James II is ruler of England.

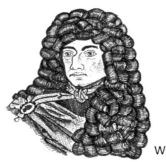

William III

In 1677 James II's daughter, Mary, marries her Dutch cousin, William of Orange. 1689 observes Mary and her husband overthrow James and they take the throne and rule jointly as William III and Mary II. The whispers around court and indeed Europe suggest that William has a fancy for young men; his lack of interest in his mistresses arouses the wagging tongues of his enemies. William's favourites are said to be William Bentinck and Arnold van Keppel. Bentinck and the king have a strong devotion to one another; Bentinck is decorated with the titles of Baron Cirencester, Viscount Woodstock and Earl of Portland however Bentinck becomes jealous of van Keppel who is bestowed the titles of Viscount Bury, Baron Ashford and Earl of Albemarle. Mary who has lived miserably having lost many children and never knowing the joys of motherhood dies in 1694, and William rules alone while van Keppel is gifted much land and money with the disapproval of Parliament. He remains close to William in his final years; he is given the honour of becoming a Knight of the Garter two years before William's death.

18th Century

It is this century that is one of the most interesting in the persecution of homosexuality. In 1721 Catherina Margaretha Linck is executed in Germany for female homosexuality. The Dutch Republic carries out the brutal and ruthless persecution of same-sex couples and those who engage in its activities. The year 1779 sees Thomas Jefferson arrange an outline summary of Virginia's criminal statute, visualising that men who practice homosexual activity will be castrated and women will have a hole, half an inch in diameter bore into the cartilage of their nose. In the late 1700s, Jeremy Bentham, a philosopher and social reformer who believes in equal rights for both men and women, becomes one of the first to call for the decriminalisation of homosexual relationships in England. The Kingdom of Prussia also make a huge leap as they abolish the death penalty for homosexuality.

Meanwhile back in Britain... again...

Queen Anne is the sister to the late Mary II and daughter of over-thrown monarch James II. It's 1702 and Anne ascends the throne after the death of her brother-in-law, William III. Anne is said to have relationships with ladies of her court and they are more than just platonic, it is said that they are sexual relationships and these continue until the end of her reign in 1714.

19th Century

It is during this century that the word 'asexual' is coined for the first time to describe a person who has no particular interest in sexual activities or an attraction to a specific gender. It sees Russia, Poland and the German Empire criminalise same sex activity whilst Argentina, Brazil, Empire of Japan, Guatemala, Mexico, Portugal, San Morino and Turkey decriminalise it.

It is in 1836 that Great Britain witnesses the last execution for homosexuality and in 1861 the law is amended to officially discard the death penalty and adjusted to imprisonment, which carries a term of anywhere from ten years to life.

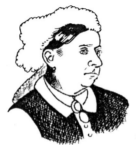

Queen Victoria

In 1886, Queen Victoria (who is not gay – well a change is as good as a rest) grants the Criminal Law Amendment Act 1885 which forbids same sex relationships between men, however nothing is mentioned about women (it is said that no-one would dare inform the Queen how two women could have carnal relations – she would certainly not be amused). Also, in this year Portugal recriminalise homosexuality after it was decriminalised in 1852.

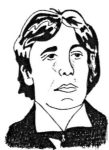

Oscar Wilde

1895 becomes the year that one of the most dishonourable trials of the century hits Queen Victoria's England. British playwright and poet Oscar Wilde is charged and tried for "gross indecency" with other men. He is convicted under the Criminal Law Amendment Act 1885, the same law Queen Victoria gave Royal Assent, and he is sentenced to two years in prison with hard labour. He dies impoverished in 1900.

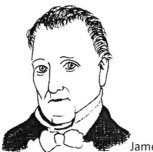

James Buchanan

It is alleged that James Buchanan, the 15th President of United States of America is also gay, and that he was romantically involved with William Rufus King - the pair shared a home together fifteen years previous to

Buchanan's term in office.   King decides to parts company with Buchanan and he goes on to become Vice President of the United States and dies forty-five days later, making him the shortest serving Vice President.   Buchanan takes up office in 1857 and will remain President until 1861.

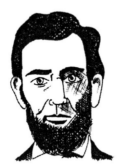

Abraham Lincoln

The same allegation also falls on Abraham Lincoln, the 16th US President whose term in office begins in 1861, it is said that he shares his bed with other men.   In Russia, Tchaikovsky the great composer speaks openly about his suppressed homosexual feelings in letters.   During his life he marries but still seeks solace with other homosexual men and he and his wife have no children.

20th Century

The turn of the 20th Century sees the word faggot printed for the first time in a publication in the United States of America in a way to demoralise those who are homosexual.

1920s

The word 'gay' is spoken for the first time in connection with homosexuality in 1920. The remaining decade of the Roaring Twenties witnesses the decriminalisation of homosexual acts in the USSR, Panama, Paraguay and Peru. Radclyffe Hall publishes 'The Well of Loneliness' which brings the subject of homosexuality to the forefront of society.

Gay people in Germany enjoy a higher level of freedom and acceptance until the Nazi regime come into force.

1930s

In 1932 Poland decriminalises homosexuality after making it illegal in 1835 and Denmark, Philippines and Uruguay follow in legalising the act. The USSR cannot seem to make up its mind as it decriminalises homosexuality in 1932 and then recriminalise it in 1933. During this time it is suggested that Eleanor Roosevelt, the wife of 32nd US President, Franklin D. Roosevelt, has a long standing relationship with a woman, a US journalist and they both have a very close relationship. Franklin is held in much regard as he serves four terms in office during his career.

In Nazi Germany people are fleeing Germany as a large purge breaks out to capture anyone who is gay, lesbian and bi-sexual. Those who are captured, if not murdered are sent to the concentration camps. The Gestapo are brought in so that names and addresses can be compiled of all homosexuals in order to guarantee maximum elimination. Those who are homosexual, once caught are not treated as abysmally as the Jewish. Gay men are forced to change their sexual orientation in order to become part of the "Master Race" and those who fail are sent to the camp, and many hundreds of gay men are castrated.

The gay men that are sent to the concentration camps are treated appallingly. They are assigned the most dangerous and punishing work, many are beaten to death by soldiers and straight prisoners alike. They are used as shooting targets for soldiers and as medical experiments for doctors in order to locate the 'gay gene' so that future generations might be cured. Many gay men die through these experiments; some extreme methods of 'curing' homosexuality come in the form of electric-shock treatment.

1940s

In quick succession during the 1940s Iceland, Switzerland, Sweden and Suriname legalise homosexuality. Switzerland and Sweden both proclaim that the age of consent for same sex relationships is 20. Portugal once again is unsure which side it's batting for as it decriminalises the act in 1945 which is the second time they have done this in their history. 1948 sees Poland set the age of 15 as the proper age of consent of homosexual and heterosexual sex.

1950s

Greece, who at the beginning of time had very large appetites for homosexual activity, decriminalise homosexuality in 1951 and Thailand then follows. This decade sees the first ever gender reassignment surgery performed taking someone from male to female, this creates a worldwide commotion. Psychologist Evelyn Hooker writes a study viewing homosexual males as well adjusted as heterosexual males (and it is this report that assists in the removal of homosexuality from the handbook of disorders belonging to the American Psychiatric Association).

In 1954 whilst working as a journalist for the British newspaper, The Daily Mail, Peter Wildeblood is sentenced to eighteen months imprisonment for homosexual relations with other men. In front of the court he confesses to being gay – this brings homosexuality to the public attention. This scandal sees the need for the Wolfenden Committee, a committee headed by Lord Wolfenden to investigate the need to change how homosexual behaviour is outlawed. The committee come to the conclusion that the United Kingdom should decriminalise homosexual relations between consenting adults. The ironic thing of all is Lord Wolfenden's son, Jeremy, is in fact gay himself.

1960s

In 1961 Hungary and Czechoslovakia decriminalise homosexuality and Illinois is the first state in the US to abolish homosexuality from its criminal code. Meanwhile in the same year the Vatican declares that those who are "affected by the perverse inclination" of homosexuality should be prohibited from taking religious vows, and neither can they be appointed within the Roman Catholic Church (which is pretty ironic because what we don't know in 1961 but discover as we move in to the

28

21st Century is that some Catholic priests who preach this nonsense are in fact indulging their unnatural behaviours through abusing young, innocent children).

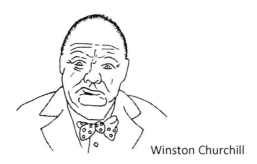
Winston Churchill

1965 sees the death of one of Great Britain's most loved figure heads, Winston Churchill. It is alleged that during Churchill's lifetime he had a sexual encounter with Welsh born entertainer, Ivor Novello, who was a well-known for his homosexual tendencies and famous for his string of fascinating relationships.

Towards the end of the 1960s the Republic of Chad and Bulgaria both decriminalise homosexuality and East Germany do the same and the age of consent is set at 18.

1970s

The Gay Liberation Day March and The Gay Freedom Day March are held in New York and Los Angeles in 1970. A year later and homosexuality is decriminalised in Austria, Costa Rica and Finland; and the states of Colorado and Oregon abolish the homosexuality laws. Idaho follows suit but then re-instates the law due to the outrage from the Mormon and Catholic churches. The Netherlands changes the homosexual age of consent to be the same as the heterosexual age of consent, 16.

As the world heads into the 1980s the view of those who indentify as being gay, lesbian, bi-sexual and transgender changes drastically – for the better.

Sweden becomes the first country to allow transsexuals who have undergone gender reassignment surgery to get their new assigned gender recognised on their personal documentation. Panama is the second country to follow in this decision.

Hawaii, Malta, Norway, South Australia, Cuba, Spain, Croatia, Montenegro, Slovenia and Vojvodina all legalise homosexuality and West Germany reduces the age of consent for homosexuals to 18. A GLBT telephone helpline is introduced to the United Kingdom – thank you Alexander Graham Bell without whom this would not be possible – he was not gay but still a great man.

The 1970's is also when the rainbow flag is used for the first time to represent the GLBT community. Finally people can express their true colours.

1980s

This decade will also see major transformations around the world starting in the United States of America, when the United States Democratic Party give their full support towards gay rights and David McReynolds is the first gay candidate to run for President of the United States. Scotland and Guernsey decriminalise homosexuality as do Northern Ireland; however they need a lot more persuading before doing so. Laguna Beach, California elects their first openly gay mayor. Reverend Jerry Falwell of the United States has the clever idea of labelling AIDS the "gay plague", how very charitable of him.

Towards the end of this decade Western Australia and Liechtenstein legalise gay relationships whilst Denmark go a step further to become the first country to allow civil partnerships for same sex couples. This will allows same sex couples the same rights as straight couples yet the marriages cannot take place in a Church and adoption is prohibited.

Another significant event happens during this decade when Hollywood heart throb Rock Hudson dies of AIDS. He is the classic leading man who has starred in a string of romantic comedies with leading lady, Doris Day. His sexuality is something that is kept private and very few people know he is gay until the revelation comes that he is suffering from AIDS. At first it is announced that he is suffering cancer, and then a press release reveals he has AIDS and is the result of having infected blood following a blood transfusion. Rock Hudson is the first prolific celebrity to die of AIDS, and after hearing of his death the House of Representatives in the US agree to double the amount of funds for AIDS research for the following year, 1986.

1990s

The last decade of the 20th Century will see equality and acceptance toward the GLBT community grow from strength to strength. Albania, Belarus, Bermuda, Cyprus, Estonia, Gibraltar, Isle of Man, Jersey, Latvia, Lithuania, Macedonia, Moldova, Romania, Russia, Serbia, South Africa and Ukraine legalise same sex relationships and Nicaragua takes a step back and recriminalise homosexuality.

Paragraph 175, a stipulation of the German Criminal Code created in 1871 which declares that acts between men to be illegal, is retracted in Germany. Canada awards refugee status to those who fear for their lives in their home country for being homosexual.

As events move rapidly in favour of the GLBT communities with more countries allowing civil partnerships, this decade sees the murder of individuals because of their sexual orientation. Some lives are ended through suicide.

1990 and Justin Fashanu who is the United Kingdom's first £1,000,000 black footballer comes out as being gay. He, like other sporting heroes is encouraged to keep his homosexuality under wraps from the public but not heeding this advice he comes out to the nation. This revelation is met with a surge of media interest, his career as a sporting hero is over as no football club wants to touch him. Whilst holidaying in 1998 at his home in the US, allegations are made by a seventeen year old male that suggest that Fashanu sexually assaulted him. After being quizzed by police he returns home to England, not long after he breaks into a garage and hangs himself leaving a suicide note expressing his innocence and stating that the sex was consensual. His note goes on to say that he has been presumed guilty when in fact innocent. An inquest into his death records a verdict of suicide. It is announced after Fashanu's death that there are no charges in regards to the earlier allegation due to lack of evidence.

21st Century

So here we are in modern day history. We have reached yet another millennium, opened copious amounts of champagne and sung Old Lang Syne to welcome in the New Year, the new millennium.

In the United Kingdom we witness the ban preventing gay and lesbian's serving in the armed forces eliminated and the age of consent for consensual sex equalised.

In the rest of the world, Azerbaijan and Georgia which are the former states of USSR decriminalise homosexuality as does Armenia, Cape Verde, China, Gabon, India, Marshall Islands, Nicaragua and Panama. Belize decides to recriminalise the act in 2003 and the year before this Sweden is the first country to allow gay couples to legally adopt.

The Bundestag, the German Parliament release an official apology to the gay and lesbian victims who were persecuted under Nazi Germany and for harm caused to homosexual people up to 1969.

Section 28, a controversial addition to the United Kingdom's Local Government Act 1986 that will not promote homosexuality in any way is revoked in Scotland first, then England and Wales allowing freedom for teachers and all other professionals employed by the government to discuss homosexuality without fear of breaking the law. It was yet another law brought in by politicians... and we all know they are strictly heterosexual. You will never see them standing at the front gates of their family home with their wife at their side apologising for an indiscretion with a male prostitute, for example.

2010

This is a hugely important decade as it sees the release of Closets Are For Clothes for the everyday person on the street who might not feel at ease with what they have been given. It allows the reader to take a brief step back in time to witness the great people who brought us to where we are now.

We don't know of the wonderful people who brought about the right for same sex couples to adopt in Sweden, or the people who pushed and fought for Portugal to legalise homosexuality, only for them to decriminalise it a further twice... third time really is lucky. These people all around the world who have positively helped our cause cannot all be listed here, some are in fact anonymous to a lot of us – but we salute you.

If being gay means that we share something with others who are gay then we are in very good company, with rulers of great nations and empires; poets, composers and political heroes; scientists, inventors and artists; and with everyday folk like you and me who just want to do good in the world.

It seems as if religion has always played a huge part in the criminalisation and decriminalisation for homosexuality. It can be hard to juggle faith and the matters of the heart and in a moment we will look how these can be resolved successfully.

We have moved on magnificently since the dawn of time, but how far have we really moved on when we know that there most definitely are football legends that are in the United Kingdom Premiership who are gay and so terrified that they remain in the closet? And the saddest thing of all is they are encouraged to stay there.

CHAPTER THREE

Religion & Beliefs

It is crucial to mention this subject early on as I and so many people and maybe you, are governed by their faith and sometimes follow what their religious readings advocate or condemn instead of their hearts. Or indeed there may be conflict in what your scriptures dictate. If you do not have any religious beliefs then feel free to skip this section. If you wish to read on it may even help you in future situations with a friend or a family member who might have a dilemma resulting in them being torn between their faith and their heart. As a Christian follower, I have written from this perspective, many other religions and beliefs have their own views on homosexuality, but as they are so wide and varied, I urge you to carry out your own research, using your preferred texts or the internet. But be aware that in many countries around the world, homosexuality is dealt with harshly - at the extreme end, life imprisonment or even death.

LIZ BOWMAN'S STORY

"I was eleven years old and living in New Orleans when I started to have really strong feelings for my best friend, who was female. As I got older I found that I was interested in both sexes. I always knew how I felt about both men and women, but I never told anyone until I was thirteen, when I confided in a friend. This information was overheard and spread throughout my school and small hometown. My grandmother, with whom I lived with at the time, stopped talking to me for weeks and I was threatened with expulsion from my Catholic School if I continued to discuss it.

The Principal and Vice-Principal arranged a meeting with my grandmother and I. They instructed me to refrain from discussing my sexuality on school grounds, and that if I didn't I would be "requested to return to the public education system". So during my time there, I did in fact keep my mouth shut and my biggest regret was not standing up for myself, and still is. I have made my peace since then.

At fourteen, I identified as bi-sexual. I was constantly teased at school, I was followed home, taunted, had trash thrown at me, and the list goes on. However I was bullied for having a bi-sexual mother. As I think back to those days I do my best to remember the people who were kind to me in life.

When I came out it was much easier to talk about who I was, that is once I was able to find a social group that accepted who I was. Once I had left my Catholic School and went back to Public School, although at times the education was lacking, my friends were the best possible thing to happen to me.

When I told my parents, I knew it wouldn't be a big deal. Their responses, verbatim, were, "Okay?" After they had spent years attending the Rocky Horror Picture Show, I didn't expect much less from them, but to me it was the best response I could have received. My parents love me for the kind, loving, considerate person that I am and that is all that matters.

Being bi-sexual is just a part of who I am. I don't think I could have kept it suppressed inside. Coming out was the best thing I have done and the most difficult. It turned out much better than I thought. Afterwards I felt as if I belonged somewhere on this planet that seems hell bent on keeping all rights from people whose sexual orientation was a little different.

I consider my first serious relationship to be when I was fifteen; I dated a guy in High School for almost a year. I dated a few women here and there after we broke up, but never really landed in a solid stable relationship with any of them unfortunately, but there were a few hopefuls. Having had these experiences I learned that homosexuality has never been a problem for me. However, because a lot of my extended family is Catholic, there are topics that I feel I can't broach in family settings, opinions I'd like to state that must be silenced. I think on the whole, it's a small price to pay for civility in the family.

36

My journey has taken its toll however. I did suffer from depression for a long time after, mostly just from being surrounded by ignorance about homosexuality. It all changed in my senior year when I started meeting more open-minded people. Since moving to Seattle, that number of people just keeps growing and growing.

I have met some great friends whilst out on the scene. There is so much about the gay scene that I enjoy, the freedom to be oneself and to meet new and exciting people who don't judge me for my sexuality. It is only a small part of who I am. As long as the gay scene has adequate security to protect against violence and dangerous drug use then it can be a fantastic experience. I can thankfully say that the only bad experience I have had on the gay scene was being offered ecstasy on the dance floor. I like so many people know my own mind so I declined politely.

Today, I'm in a serious committed relationship (with a man) and have been for the last two years. We're not married yet, but our friends and family members have all asked us when we're going to tie the knot. Personally I don't think I could possibly take part in a tradition that so blatantly excludes such a large percentage of tax-paying Americans. So my answer is very often, "Not until everyone can marry". If it ever came down to it and we decided that we really did want to get married, I would only want the same rights given to gay and lesbian couples entering a civil union. If they can't be recognised nationwide, why do I deserve that right just because I want to marry a man?"

From The Beginning

Okay, let's keep this bit simple and not too theological.

The Holy Bible says that in the beginning, God made Heaven & Earth, the Earth was without form and void, darkness was upon the face of the deep; the Spirit of God was moving over the face of the waters. God said, "Let there be light"; and there was light. God saw that the light was good; so God separated the light from the darkness. God called the light Day, the darkness he called Night.

According to Genesis, the book within the Holy Bible, not the rock group, God went on to create vegetation, the animal kingdom and then mankind. Oh yeah and a tricky health conscious little serpent that made innocent bystanders eat fruit.

God created a man who was to be known as Adam. God put Adam under a deep sleep; whilst Adam slept God removed one of Adams ribs from which he created a woman, which Adam named Eve.

This section will not be a religious teaching but just a glimpse at how the Christian faith views homosexuality. It doesn't matter what your faith or religious beliefs are, if you are gay and troubled by your sexuality with regard to maintaining your faith, this book will help you realise that you are not a bad person and that you can keep your faith and your sexuality and still be true to yourself. Moreover some would agree they go hand in hand.

I'm sure you're familiar with the colloquialism that God created Adam and Eve, not Adam and Steve or Amanda and Eve. The Old Testament was written over 3,500 years ago and it wasn't actually written by God, in fact it wasn't written by just one person, it is a collection of stories and observations documented by many people through that period in history. That is why, if you actually read The Bible, whilst authoritative in its field there are many contradictory opinions. It was written by many people's different interpretation of events, for example have you ever watched a movie or read a book and discussed it with others who have also seen or read it and wondered if you had actually seen or read the same thing. As individuals we delete and distort information in order to make sense of it, we make our own version of events, so don't take every word quite literally. If we use The Bible or any other theological scriptures as an overview and live by them, show respect and tolerance to others for whom they are, then we would live in a much better world (in my humble opinion).

I come from a Christian family, we are not dedicated Church attendees, we believe in God and we say our prayers before bed, and it is not something we talk about that often, it's just there and a part of us. I have been raised to respect others and be kind to my fellow man (or

38

woman) and I do not restrict this to Sundays or Christian holidays – it is how I live my life. I beat myself up for many years about being gay and a Christian. I considered myself to be a 'sinful creature' that should make the big decision between God and my sexuality. I then had the light bulb realisation that *God* made *me* therefore I was meant to be gay. As soon as I realised this I became a lot more comfortable with myself and my place in the world. I didn't need to choose, I could have both and that is what I have. And it's fab thank you very much!

I made a pact with God growing up that I would be a good person and I would treat people as I wanted my family members to be treated. I would live by the 10 Commandments; although I was gay I would live my life honestly without bringing shame on myself or my family. So far, I have kept my side of things and look forward to continuing on this road.

Remember Who Made Whom

For ease of reference when I refer to God, consider it my referral to your God, or God as you understand Him - your higher power or your spiritual connection. All roads lead the same way.

What we must remember is that our God, no matter what your culture or faith, made us who and what we are. It is not a case that God made us and then 'we made ourselves gay', our sexuality was decided for us before we entered this world. Many believe that homosexuality is a choice or something a person can influence through neglect or by an older gay role model. There are many who believe that God wished for all human life form to be heterosexual, as we were made in his image, to be anything other than this means that we are sinners, living unclean and immoral lives and being intentionally disobedient. You will not go far wrong if you decide that you will live by the good things your religion has to say, for Christians it would be the 10 Commandments. I say just be a good person - when you meet people make it your objective to leave them a bit happier than before you met them, be honest and true to yourself.

What The Scriptures Say

I do not want you to get too weighed down here with religious teachings, nevertheless when you are in a dilemma that results in you being torn between your feelings and religion; it is natural to wonder what your Bible says. Can people be a good believer or disciple and still be gay? This is immensely difficult for anyone who has a strong faith and is battling the feelings of being gay, lesbian or bi-sexual, when most faiths consider homosexuality a sin against their higher power.

In The Holy Bible there are only two books named after women, Esther and Ruth. Esther recounts the tale of a Jewish woman who became Queen of Persia and saved her people from obliteration by confessing to the King - her husband that she was Jewish. The book of Ruth tells the story of two women whose love and support for one another helps them through difficult times. These two books contain influential messages for gay, lesbian, and bi-sexual people, however the story of Ruth raises the question of whether two people of the same sex can live in a devoted, loving relationship with the blessing of God.

The book of Genesis describes Adam's feelings for Eve as follows:

"Therefore shall a man leave his father and his mother, and shall clave unto his wife: and they shall be one flesh". Genesis 2:24

The similar wording is used in the book of Ruth to describe Ruth's feeling for Naomi. In this book her feelings are celebrated, not damned.

"And they lifted up their voice, and wept again: and Orpah kissed her mother in law; but Ruth clave unto her". Ruth 1:14

Ruth's vow to Naomi has been used to exemplify the true meaning of the marriage covenant. This passage is often read at Christian marriage ceremonies and in sermons to demonstrate the ideal love and bond a couple should have for each another. These words were spoken by one woman to another; therefore it might actually give us an indication of how God sees same-sex relationships.

However here are a few of the passages that mention homosexuality within The Holy Bible.

"Do you not know that the wicked will not inherit the kingdom of God? Do not be deceived: Neither the sexually immoral nor idolaters nor adulterers nor male prostitutes nor homosexual offenders nor thieves nor the greedy nor drunkards nor slanderers nor swindlers will inherit the kingdom of God". 1 Corinthians 6:9-10

"Do not lie with a man as one lies with a woman; that is detestable". Leviticus 18:22

"No temptation has seized you except what is common to man. And god is faithful; he will not let you be tempted beyond what you can bear. But when you are tempted he will also provide a way out so that you can stand up under it". 1 Corinthians 10:13

Should you wish to go and do your own research of The Holy Bible then you will find references to homosexuality in the following books: Genesis, Leviticus, 1 Samuel, 2 Samuel, 1 Kings, 2 Kings, Isaiah, Daniel, Joel, 1 Corinthians, Matthew, Luke and Jude. I recommend you might look at the website **www.WouldJesusDiscriminate.com** as this is an uplifting website for Christians who might be in turmoil regarding their religion and homosexuality.

Please also remember there are also passages within The Holy Bible that carry messages that are similar to the following:

"For God so loved the world that He gave His one and only Son so that whosoever believes in Him will not perish but have everlasting life". John 3:16

The Circle Of Life

Looking at the bigger picture, research has shown that homosexuality exists in the animal kingdom too. Animals also go through the same activities of bonding, affection, courtship, sex and parenting. There are many mammals, birds, fish, reptiles, amphibians and insects that display homosexual behaviour. It is foolish to think that the animal kingdom is exclusively straight. It might have escaped your notice that the mighty King of the Jungle, the Lion also has gay relationships; the males of the pride will become affectionate until they come across a female pride. It is not just males that look to their own sex for fulfilment; this also extends to female animals that are in long lasting same sex relationships. In these relationships they will live contented by setting up a home with a female partner and raising their young without any assistance from any males of that species.

Civil Ceremonies & Celebrations

Marriages are performed differently across the many faiths, cultures and religions but in theory they all have the same thing in common which is the joining of two people in matrimony. Should marriage be an exclusive religious celebration for heterosexuals only?

We have come a long way since we inhabited caves, clubbed women over the head and dragged them back to our dwellings by their hair, after wrestling Woolly Mammoths and Sabre Tooth Tigers. Surely in this day and age those who are in same sex relationships should be allowed to celebrate the love they have for one another and be allowed to share their lives in peace and without fear of sin. Of course we should – and we are getting there.

The Day Of Judgement

George Herbert wrote in 1651 "Whose house is of glass must not throw stones at another", how true yet people do don't they? You cannot change people's opinions of you, the only thing that you can do is live your life in the only way you know how and that is by making sure you are happy, healthy and safe. Being labelled as 'gay' can be weighty indeed, there is more to you than being gay, bi-sexual or transgendered. Having a good heart, being a good person and treating others with kindness and respect will take you further in life than anything else. It hasn't done me or any of those wonderful people I choose to surround myself with, both straight and gay, any harm – quite the contrary in

42

fact.   Make it a point not to suffer fools gladly, learn from your mistakes, and wise up with every lesson.   Get into the habit of surrounding yourself with people that enrich your life and block out those things that do the opposite.   You might be thinking that this is the wrong thing to do, however I have had to do this to survive, it has become the only way that I can function.   This goes for anyone, gay, straight or otherwise.

On the day of judgement do you think that you will be condemned to Hell for loving, cherishing and caring for someone just because they were born as the same gender as you?   If we worried about what others thought of us or what we believe our religion says about us then we would all remain lonely and isolated from the rest of the world meaning we would live and die alone, don't you think?   I don't believe for one moment that our God would want us to be unhappy and alone in the world.   Do you?

Condemned To Hell

Whilst I was growing up I thought I would be condemned to Hell for my feelings; this didn't come from my parents or from anyone that cared for me.   I picked it up from the internet and through what others in society said, do I believe it now?   No.   Am I right to not believe it now?   Absolutely.

I made the conscious decision early on in my life that I was going to remain celibate; I had seen that I didn't want to live a life of falling out of one bed into another like my friend, Matt.   I am not saying it was wrong as it was their choice, both parties were consenting and they both knew the score, I just knew it wasn't for me nor am I preaching to you.   A large part for me making this decision was based on the fact that if I stayed celibate then I wouldn't offend God and I could live with my conscious.   I thought that I would be a long time in Hell suffering eternal damnation as opposed to the small amount of time I would be on this Earth even if I did live my three score years and ten.   I did have a light bulb moment, a mini euphoria to call my own where everything fell into place.   I realised I could have both as long as I could live with my conscience.   Secretly I didn't think I would find a man that would love me for me, and until I had found him I would stay celibate so I had got used to that fact.

It has always been said that those who are evil are condemned to Hell; does this apply to those who are attracted to people of the same sex? You might not see it now but you will one day have a euphoric moment to call your own and you will see how absurd it is to think that your God does not love you, right now it is very real and very scary when you believe you have been condemned from the start but you haven't. Trust me. You hold the key to this place, undo the lock, open the door and walk out; you will see the bigger picture I promise you.

How To Be Gay And Still Have Your God

It is easy to merge your sexuality and your religion; you will know when you have done it successfully as your happiness will be the result. You might encounter obstacles such as living with a family who have opinions of homosexuality based on their religious beliefs. There are ways to keep God and to remain true to yourself. That is the holiest of all Grails

- Take The Teachings In Context

Extract the things that make you feel good from your religious books, take the teachings and stories that appeal to you most and centre your attention on them. That is not to say the rest is redundant.

- Build Your Own Place Of Worship

God is all around us, you do not need to go to a Church, Mosque, Mandir, Synagogue, Gurdwara or any other place of worship if you do not feel that it is right for you. You don't have to visit these places of worship to show your love for your God or your faith. You can talk to God in the privacy of your own home. That said, there are gay and lesbian ministers.

- Surround Yourself With Like Minded People

Many gay people who battle with the conflict of their faith and their sexuality feel self-hatred, which in turn has forced them to lose their faith, caused breakdowns or even suicide. There are religious groups out there that respect your sexuality and allow you to follow your faith, just try a few searches using an online search engine. Please do your research on any of the groups you find. You will need to do your homework.

KEVIN MYNATT'S STORY

"I first remember that I felt an outsider from all the other kids in my class when I was about five years old; I noticed I liked boys and not girls and always questioned whether this was right. I did not know what gay was at the time so I was very confused.

I was brought up as a Southern Baptist, and now I am Methodist. I struggled with the fact that God would hate me because that is all I heard from the preachers. I feared going to Hell because I was such a sinner in Gods eyes. I then talked with other people and prayed a whole lot.

I was continually picked on in middle and High School, being called gay but I didn't really understand why, I knew I was different and I didn't tell anyone about my feelings. This verbal abuse would usually come from the jocks in my year and the older guys in school. I was always so scared to even say I was gay in High School for fear I would be beaten up or maybe even killed for being different; I was living in rural North West Alabama at the time.

I was always very mindful about my coming out and I feared having to come out of the closet, living in a part of the world were homosexuality was not accepted, but misunderstood. I was nineteen when I first told a female friend of mine on the phone. She said "I already knew I was just waiting for you to tell me". This was the best response I could have received. I then decided to come out to my friends and never had anyone turn their back on me. I was really surprised by this being in a small town and all, but all I got was support. The first family member I told that I was gay was my younger sister. She was cool with it, ironically she was gay herself but had not told me. I came home at Christmas break to have my mother ask me if I was gay, I replied "Yes". She said, "Well your sister came home the other day and said, Mom, Kevin is gay (long pause) and so am I!" So my sister did all the hard work for me. Later on, my aunt outted me and my sister to my dad's side of the family. She told everyone she was inviting my partner and my sister's partner to Christmas dinner and if they did not like it they did not have to come.

I am glad to say that I have always had positive experiences. Mom and Dad neither agree with it, but they tell me they still love me and for me that is all that matters. I felt liberated and felt a big weight was lifted just from them knowing the real me. It is very good to not live a lie anymore. My parents and I are still very close. My father at first would not talk to my sister and I, he removed us from his will, and encouraged his family not to talk to us both. Of course his family ignored his requests but it hurt us both when this happened. Mom and Dad say it is a choice, not what God wants, but they love us.

Coming out was the best thing I have ever done and my sister would say the same. When I was pushed to the back of the closet I felt so alone and wanted to kill myself. I was happy to end it all, I was always so depressed, now I can talk to any of my friends and know I am loved and that they do not judge me.

My first sexual experience came when I was twenty and the guy in question was thirty-two and he was my boss at work. My first relationship was at the age of twenty-three; he was living life as a straight gay and married.

My advice to anyone coming out is to surround yourself with people that love you for who you are. This is what I did and still do today. I get frustrated that gay people do not have the same rights as heterosexuals, I see this happen in society and that aggravates me. I never really have had anyone say anything negative, I know that I have been lucky but I have had my fair share of pain growing up which more than makes up

46

for it. I was very suicidal before coming out. I have gone to therapy, but it was thanks to my friends as they are the ones who really helped me through it.

I am not sure if the scene differs here to other states and countries but in my opinion there are several gay scenes. In Knoxville where I live the gay community is separated. You have your twinks, bears, transgender, lesbian and bi-sexual in their individual groups. There is a lot of promiscuous behaviour, drugs, alcoholism and depression and it saddens me to say it.

I am at peace with myself, the world and all its inhabitants. Now I feel that God does not make mistakes, so I cannot be a mistake. God says "Thou shall not judge" and I think perhaps we are all a little guilty of that sometimes. I have been shown in scripture where it says other things that most Christians overlook about God's love and tolerance of others. I do believe and know God loves me and everyone else on this earth no matter what.

I have not found my soul mate yet and I am not looking, when it happens it will happen. I am terminally single, that is what I tell my friends or anyone who asks. I will meet Mr. Right one day but for now he eludes me".

CHAPTER FOUR

I'm Coming Out... I Want The World To Know

What Is Coming Out All About?

The process of coming out allows you to become a whole person, when the day comes that you decide to come out it will be one of the most difficult things you will ever do. There is a huge upside to this; it will also be the greatest thing you will ever do. When you hide your sexuality and your true feelings it requires a lot of mental and emotional effort. When you come out you are lifting the barriers and you will enjoy expressing the person you really are, what you really feel and how you wish to live your new life. Please only do this when you are ready: Do not get pressured into coming out, it should be done in your own good time.

When you think about coming out, you will imagine yourself having to tell all your friends and family about your innermost feelings. It is perfectly fine that you feel vulnerable at this point. It's a good thing; it's your body's defences working overtime to make sure that you understand the seriousness of this and are equipped to deal with any reactions. Before taking the brave step of telling others about your feelings, the first thing you will need to do is start accepting your own sexuality, begin to love yourself from within so you can live a well rounded, happy and healthy life. What I am trying to say is that you should be comfortable with yourself first so that others can be comfortable with you too.

The Best Thing You'll Ever Do

You will know inside when it is the right time to come out. I am not alone when I say it is the best thing I have ever done, to say that a huge weight had been lifted is an understatement. I told my mother and father over the phone whilst they were living in South Africa! They spent five years out there with my dad's job. I could not even say the word gay so instead I copped out and told them I was like my friend whom they both knew was gay. It is a big step, you are coming to terms with accepting yourself and you are expecting others to do the same. Once you have come out you immediately start a better life.

Be honest with yourself and then honest with those around, especially the ones you love and those who love you. It is hard and once you have done it, you'll never look back and then you will wonder what you were worried about after all. I can't tell you how you will feel as we are all different, our situations are different. I will tell you of my experience of coming out – no holds barred.

If you are lucky enough to have understanding parents, siblings, friends and family it will bring you closer. After coming out you will need to take time for them to get to know the real you, it will be time to show people the happier, more confident person who has a restored high level of self-esteem. The secrets you hold onto before coming out are pushed so deep down within you it is hard to let them come to the surface, you will then feel better and even sleep better, there is nothing more to worry about. It is normal to feel guarded, again this is a survival technique, you will learn to become less guarded when people know the real you.

When I first went on the gay scene I hadn't come out. I told people I wasn't gay. At that time I wasn't prepared to come to terms with the fact I was gay. I knew at that time I didn't want to tell people I was bi-sexual when I knew full well I wasn't. I had known people who had told their parents they might be bi-sexual when they knew they were gay, they use the term bi-sexual to soften the blow to their parents as this leaves a glimmer of hope that they just might meet someone of the opposite sex. Needless to say it did not go down too well with other gay people on the scene when I told them I was not gay when they knew full well I was. It gave them ammunition, they knew, I knew but I wasn't ready to say it. I would go as far as saying they looked down their nose at me. As I think back to this time I would have to say this was fair play, I was in their club looking for sanctuary when in actual fact I was denouncing what it all stood for. That was a lesson for me; I went away and had a long hard think. I came out not long after that, not because I felt forced, but it was the wake up call that told me that enough was enough. I realised when I came out that it was easier to socialise with other gay people. There were no barriers and no secrets. When I came out and went to a bar, I put every effort into my appearance so I would not stand too far out of the crowd. I wanted people to look at me for being presentable and not to say "Girl, what are you wearing?" People at last saw the real me, those people who liked the real me remain an important part of my life, and I tell them so. Those who have not been able to accept the real me, we have parted company like adults, I do not wish them any harm, they leave me alone and I repay the favour.

That feeling of carrying a great weight of secrets weighs you down and by coming out it is suddenly lifted, one feels lighter being able to physically move around more. It is a good feeling people. Looking back I realise it was harder for me to appreciate I was gay than my parents. My biggest challenge was saying 'I am gay!' I choked, every time I attempted to say it. It does pass, where you are now isn't going to be where you are going to be forever. You will feel more at peace with yourself and those around you. You will have more energy, higher self-esteem, confidence and a sense of calm and when it all goes well; you will feel more love than you ever thought possible.

MICHAEL GUNDERSEN'S STORY

"I knew I was gay my whole life, I am being serious. I was fooling around with other boys in kindergarten, does that sound bad? I could write a book about being bullied in school, it was horrible. Even the teachers looked the other way most of the time as the other kids beat the crap out of me. It was a daily experience.

When I decided to come out it was actually no big deal emotionally, I was never confused about whether or not I was gay, only about when to come out to the world. My family had always been extremely gay friendly so I knew it wouldn't be a problem on that front. It was a

51

matter of getting the time right. Well the time came, I brought home the boy I was dating at the time, Johnny, I was fifteen years old. We were all sat around the table and I told them that we were together and what's more we were in love. Then I asked my mom to pass the ketchup.

It was better than I thought at first, but Mom and Dad knew first hand the terrible ways the world treated their gay friends and hated the thought of me being harmed in the same way. I was expecting the "are you sure it's not a phase?" speech, but it never happened. It went kind of wrong when my dad said that he had experimented with homosexuality when he was sixteen and tried to talk about his gay sexual experiences in order to be supportive, but ewwwww, that's my dad! All said and done, I was happy that it was officially out in the open. "Mom, where is the ice cream?"

I could not imagine a more wonderful, supportive family. My whole family refers to my husband as such. My retired marine elder brother, although uber heterosexual and politically conservative, is a staunch supporter of gay rights and has no problem telling homophobes where to shove it. I have heard of times when friends or acquaintances of his made disparaging remarks about me, or gay people in general, and although I am against violence, it does make me smile that he beats the crap out of them.

To me, coming out has neither been the best thing I have done or the worst, it was just a part of life.

My first relationship happened during my freshman year in High School, we were together as boyfriends until his family found out. They literally moved to another state and forbade all contact with me. It was my fault, they found my love letters to him, and his father is from a country in Africa where gays were and still are put to death. It broke my heart, and for twenty years I lived with the guilt of what had happened to him, not knowing anything, crying on occasion for the loss of him in my life and for the suffering I was sure he was going through. Wouldn't you know that thanks to FaceBook, we recently reconnected and I found out that his being found out was the best thing that ever happened to him!!!

I literally felt like the entire weight of the world was lifted from my shoulders.

I thankfully didn't suffer depression as so many others do when they have been in my situation of being attracted to the same sex. Perhaps it is because I didn't put any serious emotion behind it, it was a part of me. Other than experiencing the typical hormone laced teenage drama queen stuff there is nothing to report.

I do enjoy an occasional night out on the gay scene; parts of it are awesome, parts not so much. For example, the gay scene in Chicago and New Orleans where I have lived was really wonderful, yet where my husband and I have lived for six years now it is horrible. It depends on where you are and who is there with you.

I have been with my Mr. Right for about a decade now. We gave ourselves a ceremony here in Florida, where we had no friends because his doctors said that he would soon pass away and we couldn't wait for friends. We have been blessed, however, because doctors said that he had a 100% chance of passing away within that year, and here we are six years later. Every day is a blessing, and our bond grows stronger".

Helping Others To Come Out

Another experience that might arise when you meet a prospective partner, you may have come out and they haven't. This can be a difficult situation.

I can relate to this having had first hand experience, it is difficult and by working through it you can get through it. Andrew and I were together for two years and then I 'outted' him to my parents, he was an important part of my life and so were my parents. It is difficult when you are in a serious relationship to deny you are in a relationship, it does nothing for your self-esteem. I felt that by not being 'out' together, it was holding us back from enjoying life to the full. And I was right.

Should you find yourself in a similar situation it is natural to feel that your relationship is bound in limitations. It is even trickier when you know you have found the right person and feel stuck in these circumstances. It does hurt when you know you are so similar yet so different and with time, patience and understanding it will work itself out. If you are sure that your partner is Mr or Mrs Right then work at it as hard as you need to. If you are not willing to be patient in the early days of your relationship you may need to make some even harder decisions later on. Your future happiness will depend on doing what is right for you, and not for someone else.

The day after I came out to my parents I went into work as usual, and I told my friends and colleagues that I was gay. I found that after I came out others followed. I am not saying they decided to do this because I did, but if they accept one person, and then another, and another, they will accept you. Your family, friends and colleagues will accept you too.

Coming Out Step By Step

For the record, there is no right way to come out. You can plan as much as you like, the experience is not at all enjoyable. You should give your coming out some thought, it is important that you are comfortable and confident and you know exactly what you want to say. Planning your coming out is not as fun as planning the family barbeque, make sure that you remain in control of this process and be prepared to answer any questions that your friends or family might have. Take it step by step, don't rush it and make sure you are ready to do this.

- Coming Out To Yourself

You need to be absolutely sure that you want to live your life as a gay man or woman before you come out. You can't jump out of the closet and jump straight back in again. You need to accept yourself for what and who you are. Be forgiving towards yourself, there is nothing wrong with being gay and being an individual, everything is about you living a happy life. The end result will be having the support, love and reassurance of your friends and family: That is your desired outcome.

- Come Out To Your Friends

I came out to a friend at work in the first instance, he was also gay and we got on well together. This might be the first option, tell your friends as you know that they love you for who you are, your sexuality being neither here nor there. When they accept you, you will feel a confidence that allows you to increase the circle of people you tell. Don't be alarmed if your friends act negatively or seem to be a little different, it might be their lack of understanding and once they have had time to adjust, it will work out fine. Do not take any of the questions they ask personally, they might not get the whole gay thing and therefore have a few questions. The more you talk about it and answer their questions you will feel at ease speaking about it.

- Come Out To Your Family

Again using the same model as coming out to your friends, pick someone in the family you have a strong bond with. If they love you just the way you are they should stand by you and might even help you come out to others. It might be a sibling or a cousin; it could even be a grandparent or favourite aunt or uncle. Do not be fooled by the fact that grandparents are old therefore they do not understand what it is to be young. They were young once and had all the anxieties that you and your friends have felt, maybe even worse. You will find that they have grown up with lots of gay entertainers such as John Inman, Kenneth Williams, Frankie Howard, Wilfred Bramble and the like. These legends were successful at their craft for being quick witted, articulate and expressive characters. They were larger than life and people loved them. You only need to look on the television now at the modern day entertainers who are openly out and proud of their sexuality a freedom that was not enjoyed be their forebears.

- Come Out To The World

This is not an opportunity to announce your coming out in The Times, it is about fully committing yourself to coming out in every stage of your life by means of telling your work colleagues, the people you socialise with and the people you play football with on a Sunday. Begin by telling the people you are close to and increase the circle from there. Give them time to absorb what you have told them, they will support you.

- Come Out To The School

I have palpitations just thinking about coming out to those in school. If I can offer any advice to you, DO NOT even think about coming out at school. Should you wish to come out at school please read Chapter Twelve that discusses in great detail about bullying at school. Prepare yourself to think long and hard about who you want to come out to. Do you want everyone to know, if so is it because you want to be accepted or are you doing this for the attention. Once you are out, you can't go back in. You can always say you were lying, joking or confused, it's easy to get a label to stick, but removing it is a lot harder.

No Dramatics

The timing of coming out is all important and this is why you should choose your timing carefully. You don't want your coming out to be like a scene from your favourite soap opera. There will be no shouting or screaming in the middle of the street, no sliding down doorways and no drunken arguments. Get yourself in a comfortable place mentally, emotionally and physically, make sure there is nothing else going on.

Timing is everything and so is location. If you feel that you cannot tell them at home choose a neutral spot and no, I'm not suggesting you make a dash for the morning talk show. Make sure that your location is familiar and calming so you are relaxed.

Things To Remember When Coming Out To Your Parents

Remember, I told my parents over the phone as they were on the other side of the world. I told my mother first and then she went away and told my dad. It might be easier to tell one and gain their support to tell the other. My mother was shocked but not disappointed, she said she would never have guessed and my dad said he thought I had always been "a bit light on my loafers". That was him joking of course. My parents and I have always been extremely close; they had always been my best friends growing up. I remember telling him that he was not any less of a man for having a gay son. Thinking back it was a silly thing for me to say as he knew that already.

Be prepared for some questions, unfortunately you cannot prepare all the answers, just be honest. They may ask "How long have you known?" and "Who else knows about this?" The great thing about this book is it appeals to everyone who is touched by being different or coming to terms with someone who is different. Reading this book might actually give them a better understanding of you and the dilemmas you have faced.

After coming out many people say they wish they had done it sooner, that's exactly what I said and felt. I was twenty-one when I came out and sincerely wish I had done it sooner, which is just my personal preference, it was the right time though. It happened at that time because it was the right time for me. It will be for you, as you will see.

You may think that knowing your parents for as long as you have that you will know how they will take your news, but remember they may take it much better than you think. Many parents do discuss with their friends gay characters in society, so may not react in the negative way that you expect. You may have to prepare for the fact that the news doesn't go so well leaving you to feel that you wished you had not come out at all. If you have grown up in an environment that is openly prejudiced about gay people then there will be many that will sympathise with you as it cannot be easy feeling that you have no-where to turn. Please visit **www.ClosetsAreForClothes.co.uk** as this contains resources that will assist you with this.

In my opinion I think calling my parents to tell them about my sexuality was a cop-out but I had no choice. It was a gloomy evening in October and I wasn't seeing them until Christmas, I didn't really want to tell them then as I didn't want to ruin Christmas, should the news have taken our relationship in another direction. It could have been a very unhappy Christmas although I knew deep down they would be fine about it.

There are no rules about coming out, you can voice your coming out without having to say a word if it's too difficult to do. Should you find it difficult to speak to a parent or relative then write them a letter, something that is written from the heart. Tell them everything, the length of time you have felt the way you have, how you have felt alone and removed from the rest of the world. Explain that with their understanding, continued love and support you can finally be who you truly are and you want to live an honest and happy life that they will be very much a part of.

I have known people wait until they have moved out and gained their independence, not reliant on anyone else and have their own safe haven. Not everyone has this luxury, but remember it is all about timing, doing what is right for you.

You can now see that timing is important, it is crucial that you are in the right frame of mind. Avoid coming out at Christmas or on any other family celebration as you need to make allowances just in case it doesn't go as well as you had planned. Your common sense will tell you that you will need to take it step by step. Parents have a thing called unconditional love; they tend to be very accepting of their gay child. Don't expect to get a standing ovation from all you tell, at the end of the day you are still you, it's only a very small part of who you are. The person you are is the one who is kind, considerate, well mannered, trustworthy, honest and respectable. It may take a day or two for them to adjust; they have seen you for so many years in one way and then have to adjust to the new you.

My mother and I are close, we have always been like sisters, and she was shocked when I told her. She was not at all disappointed; she didn't cry or question God. My father, who is a man's man understood and although we have always been extremely close it has made us even closer. He has always been protective of both me and my brother, and he is even more protective towards me now as he knows there are bigots out there.

Following my phone call, my mother wrote me a note and it read:-

Dear Richard,

I am writing this letter to you for two reasons, the first one is that I wanted you to know how much your father and I love you, and the second reason I wanted you to have something to keep. So that next month, next year or even thirty years from now you will have something to fall back on, when you may doubt yourself or the life you have made for yourself.

You have always had a very close relationship with your father, the kind that even your friends have been envious of, and that bond between you both will never be broken. As for the two of us we have a relationship my friends have been envious of so always be proud of that.

You are a fine young man, and we have always been proud of you and always will be. You are the kind of son any parent would want; kind, thoughtful and loving. You really care about other people and that is rare even in the best of us. Sometimes you may feel sad and lonely, but when you do take this letter and read it. Always hold your head up high. Respect yourself and other people will respect you. You would think this letter would be the hardest for a parent to write under the circumstances, but I find it to be one of the easiest that I have ever written because I know what is right in my head and what I feel is right in my heart.

So keep this letter safe Richard, so you will always know how much we love you. Be proud, be happy and be yourself.

All my love to you,

Mam

I wish you an easy and happy coming out. If you come out and people react badly to what you have told them then re-visit the idea of writing the letter. If it is a true friend they will see the person who has always been there.

You have not hurt or maimed anyone, you are still the same person you were before coming out, and in fact you are a better person as you can now be happier, confident and more comfortable in your own skin. It is only a small part of who you are.

I believe you should try anything once, as long as you are comfortable with it apart from incest, murder and Morris Dancing.

ROBERT PITTMAN'S STORY

"I knew I was gay at about the age of eleven. You know how it is in school, I was dared to kiss a girl that liked me and I did... and nothing. I did not like it at all. This was not a pointless episode in my life because I began thinking about what it would be like to kiss a guy. I had a friend who was unbeknown to me bi-sexual, I told him how I felt about the whole kissing thing and he kissed me right there and then on the spot... and I loved it!

When it came to bullying I have had my fair share. I have been verbally and physically attacked but it was from people who didn't actually know me. When this happened no one did anything unless one of my friends was there to support me. I am ashamed to say that my family in some ways also bullied me about being gay, my mother and her side of the family treated me very badly for a couple of years because of my sexual orientation.

When I came out it was very scary and a little overwhelming, I did not know how anyone was going to react to the fact and I wasn't sure how I was going to do it. But, as I came out to more and more of my friends and got a support network I became more confident and had an easier time coming out than I had expected. I guess the secret is to start off small and gradually get bigger.   It took a very long time before I was able to tell anyone in my family, but the right time came and I sat them down and told them how I felt. Of course, they accepted me for who I am and nothing changed with a lot of them. I must admit that I first came out as being bi-sexual, just to see how they reacted, I did this to everyone even my friends. After that I came out fully and nothing changed everyone was still as supportive. Well save for my mother and her side of the family, but they came around and it's just normal now.

I must tell you that when I came out a great weight was lifted off my shoulders. It is the best thing I have ever done because I could finally be me; I liked that more than anything. I am so much stronger now and more confident, I don't recognise myself and I now know who truly matters in my life.

I had my first relationship when I was eighteen. I went out with one of my best friends from childhood he was bi-sexual, we experimented together but after a while it became obvious that he liked women more than he did men so it ended.

After this I felt totally alone but thanks to my supportive network of friends I talked and talked and got a lot of stuff out in the open and they made it quite clear that I was never going to be truly alone. I enjoy going on the gay scene with most of my friends, and for me it can be a great way to meet knew friends who understand me and that is very comforting, I thankfully have not had any bad experiences and because I am always with friends it is never a bad experience".

Using Sites To Socially Network

This might seem as if I am going off the subject matter here however it is important that we cover this subject early as networking via the internet has a profound way of how we conduct ourselves and you will see how it has become a large part of your life.

There are millions and millions of us who have overnight become accustomed to communicating via social networking websites. I'm guilty as charged. Some people are totally oblivious to the term *social networking sites* but as soon as you mention the word FaceBook, Bebo, MySpace, Twitter, Gaydar, GaydarGirls, CockBook or Girls Out Now, they know exactly what you are talking about. There are many dangers that come with sharing information on these sites and it is not always identity theft or financial fraud. It has been said that we are making ourselves vulnerable, and putting current and future professional reputations at stake by posting drunken antics, personal vendettas and comments and pictures that should remain private, in front of the world for all to see.

This is not a lecture of how to protect your identity online as this only requires common sense. You know how important it is not to post your date of birth, address and telephone numbers on the internet as this information is often used as data protection questioning amongst financial institutions such as banks and insurance companies.

Joining these groups come with warnings of remaining cautious about the content you post on these sites. It is far easier to live by the rule – 'never post anything you wouldn't want your parents to see'. It has been said that potential employers or educational institutions check social networking sites to examine a person's behaviour that might not be so apparent in an interview or examination.

There are those social networking sites that go a step further allowing the user to do more than throw a sheep at another user or send a virtual drink or birthday gift. These are websites such as Gaydar, GaydarGirls and CockBook – there are also many more should you wish to do your own research. These websites combine social networking and "dating" all in one. It is these sites that have certainly transformed the way people relate to each other on and offline. Gaydar, for example was originally created so that single gay men could hook up. Over the years it has been implicated in the downfall of politicians and celebrities alike. It is these types of websites that have been associated with sleaziness, it is where the gay community come together and meet not as friends but for sexual encounters. The user can upload photographs that really require no censoring and leave nothing to the imagination. When public figures and celebrities are found to be using these sites it hits the headlines in a big way even though they are going about their lives like all the other "normal" users. It also comes with added publicity when it involves the element of homosexuality – is it ever as much of an issue when it is done in the straight community.

Websites such as Gaydar and CockBook allow the user to enter as much or as little information as they like, the more they enter, the more they can be found to match someone else's ideal. For example if someone was in search of a Caucasian male, twenty-seven years old, with blue eyes, blonde hair, slim build, no body hair with facial stubble, who stood at 6' 1" with a cut penis, who doesn't smoke, drinks occasionally and partakes in drugs socially, practices unsafe sex, is both sexually passive and active (versatile) then they can be found. Searches can also be done using a "mile radius" method where it is possible to view men and women who live within a particular distance. Now that is advanced.

Make sure you check the terms and conditions of each social networking site you join, it is easy to create an account and upload information but sometimes it is a little harder to remove or permanently delete it.

Using the internet to network is quick and easy – and it can be fun. Do not use these websites as a crutch that substitutes normal interaction with the outside world. As you read through the book you will notice there are pertinent warnings within the chapters that relate to social networking sites like the one below. Social networking websites now feature in certain aspects of a person's life and it is important that you use them sensibly and remain the one in control.

Social Networking Site Warning:

Do not rely on FaceBook or any other website to take responsibility for your coming out. The best way to come out is by following the steps that we have already discussed. I recently witnessed a friend of a friend's coming out unfold right in front of my eyes. His name is Tom and he had a FaceBook profile that looked similar to most peoples. His relationship status said he was in a relationship with a young lady named Jennifer. He thought the best way to come out was to join the groups that were related and supportive of gay issues, he then wrote the following on Jennifer's wall:

"I am sorry Jen but I have to tell you that I am gay. It's not you it's me - I hope you can understand this difficult period in my life. I hope we can still remain friends. Love Tom X"

He then went on to update his status by saying:

"Right then guys, I think it's time I said it - I'M GAY! I would like to thank those FaceBook friends who have helped me over the last few days. I'm so glad for your kind words of support. I hope you all understand and will still be my friends. Love Tom X"

You can probably see at this moment that this was not the best way for Tom to handle the situation. Apart from humiliating his girlfriend he has lost total control of the situation. He has put the situation out there to all his friends, family, work colleagues and acquaintances – all of whom will be talking and dealing with it however they see fit. Don't drop the bombshell and wait for everyone else to pick up the pieces. Show respect to those closest to you such as your friends and family by telling them first.

DANNY BONE'S STORY

"I suppose I knew that I was gay when I got to High School. I tried to submerge my feelings towards men, but eventually I had to accept who I was. I was never really bullied at school if I am honest; I have thankfully never been the centre of anyone's hatred.

My mum is a lesbian, she came out after my dad and she parted, she had always been gay and desperately wanted me, so they split before I was born. When I decided to come out to my mates they were totally cool about it, in fact I found out later that they were taking bets behind my back as to when I would actually come out of the closet. As my mates where so good about it I presumed Mum would be cool as well especially as she knew what I was going through. This wasn't the case, at first she got really worked up about it all but with time her and her female partner have come to terms with me being bi-sexual. All is well now but I do dread telling her I have a serious boyfriend because I just know she will not like the idea, ironic don't you think?

My coming out was totally unexpected and it was all thanks to FaceBook, the social networking site – bringing people together – yeah right!? Not to put too finer point on it, I was messing around with my
64

best mate's brother, and a few things were said on FaceBook. Mum saw it; by this point I wanted to tell her but didn't know how to approach the subject. Then at Christmas, I went to the works party, and got very drunk and came home, it was then I told Mum. Probably not the best time to do it but hey when drink is involved you can take on the world.

Let's just say it went horribly wrong, she said she was disappointed that I didn't tell her whilst I was sober. We spoke about it regularly for the next few weeks and I think she has finally come around to it. I can be myself now when I am around my family and friends and this has helped me to become the person I want to be. I now know the important people in my life who love me for who I am. I am glad to say that nothing has changed really; anything that has happened has made it better. My friends have stuck by me, Mum has come around to it and the rest of the family doesn't mind either. It is the best thing I have ever done; I wouldn't have it any other way now.

I cannot 100% say that my sexuality has anything to do with it, but I did suffer mentally, I used to self harm when I was fourteen years old. I would cut myself and was sent to a Counsellor later on because of this. They said it could be down to various reasons, but I am sure it was because I was in denial about my true feelings. I overcame self harming when I met my best friend, Catherine. She helped me through a lot and we both came out around the same time so we are really close even to this day.

My first experience on the gay scene was when I visited the gay village in Manchester, all I will say is that I enjoyed it that much I am a regular visitor and I thankfully have not had a bad experience on the scene. I am careful and responsible which is how everyone should be if they want to have a good time.

I am still very young and I have a lot of life to live. I am now in my first serious(ish) relationship with a guy and I am happy to say that it is going really well – watch this space".

CHAPTER FIVE

The Gay Scene

What Is The Gay Scene?

The gay scene refers to the community where gay, lesbian, bi-sexual and transgender people socialise. It consists of gay clubs; gay pubs and gay bars, there are even gay hotels, gay restaurants and also gay holiday packages and cruises. The scene also extends to 'Gay Pride' which is a festival to celebrate our individuality, it promotes the message that it is okay to be different, it is a gift and not to be hidden. The gay scene can be a great place to socialise but only with care, this is meant with all seriousness. The scene is a great place to go since you know that other people will understand you from their experiences, you can relax and feel a part of the group. The gay scene has created its own reputation for playing the best music and creating a welcoming night scene. Many straight people also visit the gay scene for the music and the great atmosphere. There are a lot of colourful people about and you can be yourself without the worry of homophobic encounters.

When I first went on the gay scene I felt a huge sense of relief, it was reassuring to know that I was amongst people who felt and thought like me. The scene was like a refuge for me and it can be like that for most people. Our differences from regular society should be accepted instead of forcing us into isolation, being harassed or even sweeping us under the carpet. Your first time on the scene can be an overwhelming and slightly daunting experience.

The gay scene can be enjoyable as long as you remain in control. Friday and Saturday nights is when the gay scene really comes alive, a lot of people enjoy it for a number of reasons:

- The gay scene can be a lot of fun. It's not all about pubs, clubs, loud music and alcohol. There are cafes and pubs that serve coffee and good old fashioned pub lunches; they have themed nights such as tribute evenings, pub quizzes and off the wall entertainment such as drag versions of X Factor. It can be a colourful place with colourful people.

- A lot of straight people really enjoy the gay scene too; you will encounter some really grounded and un-opinionated straight groups who have fun socialising with their gay friends or just visit the venue because of the atmosphere. This will allow you to encounter a diverse range of people who understand, accept and don't judge.

- You can network and meet other like minded individuals. You might be looking for a future partner, a new friendship or just a bit of fun – just make sure you take care and do what you feel comfortable with.

- Gay pubs, clubs and bars celebrate being different and will welcome you with open arms. It can boost your confidence and show you that you are not alone.

- It can boost your self-esteem and give you a secure environment to hang out and many people build up tight groups of friends that are like second family, if that is what you are looking for. It reconfirms that there is a life after coming out, even if you visit the scene and you haven't yet come out. You have taken a big step to show that you are who you are (and what you are needs no excuses).

- You can be as openly affectionate toward your partner as straight couples can be in straight clubs and pubs.

I mentioned that the gay scene can be enjoyable as long as you remain in control; here are the negatives to the gay scene:

- I stand by everything you have just read but take it from me, if you have decided that you want to meet the love of your life then try and find them outside of the scene. I know that this contradicts everything I have just mentioned but it's true. People who visit the scene rarely go to meet Mr or Mrs Right. I am sure there have been many strong lasting relationships of couples who have met on the scene however people are usually looking for a good time and perhaps no strings fun. That is all very well as long as each consenting adult knows the situation. If you are promiscuous whilst on the scene you will find in a short space of time that you have been with everyone on the scene. Always think of the consequence of the decisions you make well in advance. Reputations are hard to build up and easy to ruin.

- The gay scene no matter how big the town or city you visit will always be quite small in relation to the size of the straight scene. When you visit the scene for the first couple of times you will be a new face, you probably will not believe this but you will be noticed, you will draw attention and people will make advances to you. The reason for this comes from the fact that many of the people on the scene have been on the scene many times, perhaps even years and before you know it you will recognise the same old faces when you visit a few times.

- The fairytale of the gay scene being all sweetness and light is just that... a fairytale. You will need to find a scene that is right for you and then you will discover some great people who will become your friends, but be warned: Like in any situation you may meet some characters whom maybe extremely skilled in using the venomous one-liners. The scene has been generalised by many people as being a bitchy place, it is usually harmless enough, there are groups who banter and throw insults to mark their territory in the same way a dog will pee against a garden wall, they are saying that they are a firm part of the scene and they are there to stay. Good for them as this happens on the straight scene too.

- Some people find the scene to be shallow, with youth, image and casual sex being coveted. People who don't fit into certain criteria can feel excluded or out of place.

- The gay scene is like anything, a moderate dose can be good for you, if consumed in excess then it can be bad. A word of caution, it can be a friendly or unfriendly place like anywhere, it is up to you to decide the parts you choose. When you have decided the role the gay scene plays in your life you can then embrace it as part of your family, as there are many who see it as a fellowship and association.

Advice When Visiting The Scene

Do not let what you have just read put you off visiting the gay scene; on the contrary it is like anything in life, there are positives and negatives. Recognise and enjoy the advantages and be wary of the disadvantages, give them a wide birth. There have been stories of young impressionable gay men visiting the scene, and becoming an easy target, they are seen as fresh blood or meat – but you are not. You have feelings and a mind of your own; remember you are in control of your reputation, your own actions and your own life.

In the UK the legal age to consume alcohol is eighteen years of age and it is twenty-one years of age in most states in the USA so remember this when visiting the scene. Don't break the law; rules are there to be adhered to. The first time on the gay scene can be quite daunting so here are a few things you can do to make sure you have a safe, enjoyable evening.

- Make arrangements for a group of your friends to visit the scene with you, the more the merrier. If you don't have a crowd of people ask a friend to join you.

- DO NOT leave drinks unattended, this advice applies when you are on the straight scene too.

- Stay in control and have rules if you are unsure of anything. For example give yourself a time to leave, if you really are enjoying it too much then you can extend it, likewise if you are not having a good time then leave, you only have to stay as long as you want to. If you are one of those people who can only have a good time after having a skin-full remember to drink sensibly and if you are not one of those people you don't have to drink at all, there are plenty of people who go out and drink bottled water, they don't need alcohol to have a great time.

- Take the evening in your stride and just be yourself. If people don't like you as you are then that is fine, you do not have to bother with those types of people, far easier to be yourself instead of trying to put on a performance.

- Be nice to people, someone may come up to speak with you and you may not necessarily find them attractive, however you should be polite and have a chat with them, you might become great friends. You should not speak exclusively to the people in the 'nice looking crowd'. A solid friendship is a stronger bond, think of the friends you have that you are not attracted to, that's why they are such good friends.

No Amateur Dramatics

The gay scene is not a stage school; avoid arguing with your partner or your rival while out partying on the scene. It is up to you how you conduct yourself while you are out in public; you will see for yourself that a lot of amateur dramatics are being performed centre stage. Many people find it necessary to play out their arguments and disagreements in full public display; this is not the best way to resolve your situation. There are those who enjoy watching these performances as much as those who are acting in them so just keep in mind what your audience will be thinking. You will be the centre of attention for sure, but is that what you want? If you have a disagreement then sort it out like adults, if you have a peccadillo before going out then do not go out until it is settled and if you quarrel whilst you're out, walk away and speak the next day when the alcohol has evaporated and you have clear minds.

ALAN'S STORY

"I knew that I was gay when I was around ten or eleven years old. I never had a problem with it, to me I was normal and what I was feeling was part and parcel of who I was. When I did realise that I was gay, I was around sixteen or seventeen years of age and wanted to jump straight onto the gay scene as soon as I could. It was around this time that I came out to my mother. We always had a great relationship and I hated hiding my feelings, lying about where I was going when I visited the pubs and clubs on the gay scene. I didn't want to hurt her by coming out but it was she who was hinting to me about my sexuality. She said she had known for sometime and she didn't care who knew, she was proud of me. My coming out went very well, and the fact that I had been honest with my mother and she knew and more importantly, accepted me and loved me, just made my forthcoming blooming onto the gay scene all that much more enjoyable.

I work on the gay scene and I love it. I perform as the fabulous drag queen, Fanny Dazzle. I definitely believe that the scene serves a purpose to those in the LGBT community. Firstly, as somewhere gay people young and old can go and relax and be themselves. They can do this without having to hide anything away or pretend to be something they are not. It is soul destroying in life to stifle who you are. We all need to be accepted, and sometimes 'being with your own kind' allows you a sense of feeling that you belong.

Secondly, the gay scene is especially important for young gay people, because when we are young we think we are the only ones. Even when we know we are not the only ones we still feel isolated and misunderstood and the gay scene can make sense of it all. It is important to keep your head and not fall for the first bloke you meet, but you can have some really good friends, if you choose them carefully.

The gay scene can be a hard place, there is backstabbing, bitching but this happens anywhere, and its all part of life's learning curve. Too many people moan about the wrongs of the gay scene however people have fought many battles to make sure we at least have one. We do have a place we can go if we choose to visit, where at the very least we don't have to hide what sometimes we feel we are forced to.

Like most people there are things I would change if I had my time again. You know the stuff, things I would not have said to people, things I wish I had said, situations that could have been left better. Knowing what I know now, if I was a teenager again with all my life in front of me and I had the choice of being gay or straight, with the life I've had, there's no way at all that I would choose to be straight. Mainly because of my sexuality, I've had an absolute hoot, a real ball. Although it hasn't always been a riotous round of laughs, in fact it has been really hard, desperate at times, I love my life and how it has turned out mainly because of the people in it.

The one mistake the over zealous people who disagree with this lifestyle think we actually choose this life. We don't! We are who we are and this life chooses us!

But the best thing about life, any life is, if we want something then we can at least try to make it happen, we are in charge of our own destiny".

You can find out more about Alan and Fanny Dazzle in Chapter Fifteen.

Create Your Own Scene

If going pubbing and clubbing is not for you then do something about it. You can either lock yourself in a dark room forever, if that's what you really want to do, but this would not be recommended as this would make for a miserable existence and no good for your mental health. Another option would be to create your own scene. You will meet other gay people outside of the scene, perhaps at work, through friends and it is surprising how many people on FaceBook who you used to go to school with come bouncing out of the closet - sometimes the ones you least suspect. Yes, they are human after all!

There are social networking sites like FaceBook and chat rooms where you can find like minded people and this should be done with caution.

When you have the World Wide Web between you and the person you are talking to things get lost in translation such as sending and receiving pictures that are not really you or them, or perhaps it is them and they accidently sent a picture that was taken twenty years ago. Do not get caught up in relying on chat rooms to get friends or relationships. It is very easy to get into that pattern of cyber-talk and many people, who are not necessarily gay, become more interested in getting to their computer to have a friendship instead of actually getting involved in the real world.

The internet is a great place to catch up on any events that might take your interest and there are masses of websites where you join groups virtually and physically. If you are an active person you could join the local football team, if you look in the right place then you might find a gay football or rugby team that meet once or twice a week. If there is not one in your area and you have enough friends, why not start your own? If you like running then join up to an existing running club or create your own. Whatever you like doing there are surely others with the same interest. Find them and become part of something, and do your research. That is what the internet is for. Please visit **www.ClosetsAreForClothes.co.uk** as this contains resources that will assist you with this.

Now, that dark room doesn't seem so appealing now, does it?

EMILY VIRGINIA'S STORY

"I knew I liked women from around the age of fifteen. I was really rather fortunate as I was never bullied for being gay. I knew others in school that were not so fortunate. I didn't have to suppress my feelings for long; I was only in the closet for about two or three months after realising my true feelings. I couldn't wait to bust out of there. I needed to say something to someone and when I told all those who were important to me; the positive reactions confirmed that I had made the right choice.

I came out by telling my nearest and dearest one at a time, I started with my best friend, then my band mates, and when it was widely

74

accepted amongst my peers I told my parents and then the family. It sounds weird now I recall the story and I told my friends and band mates before I told Mom and Dad but I was still nervous about telling people and there was safety in numbers. Well, so I thought at the time.

It went better than I could ever have thought, it wasn't a big deal or anything and no one treated me any differently either, no one made a big song and dance, in fact I actually thought there would be more excitement over it. From that moment onwards I felt a lot better being myself than keeping a secret. It doesn't matter much, but the tension of holding in a secret isn't great and now I no longer have that burden.

I have a wonderful relationship with my parents, and family, my friends have always treated me the same, some people like me even more now I can be me. It made me grow up a bit quicker too, it was certainly the most important thing I have had to do so far, but as personal experiences go, I certainly would call it my best.

I now have a girlfriend, but we're not married or anything. I love her very much though and I think our relationship will last the test of time. My girlfriend is a supporter of GLBT community and I'm not, it's not that I'm not proud of who we are or don't wish to socialise with other like minded individuals, I just like to keep my affections more private. I also have to stop her sometimes from holding my hand or hugging me too long in public because you don't know who's watching, but around friends I'm fine with it".

In Summary

The gay scene is what you make it. If your intention is to go out and have a good time where you are not harming yourself or anyone else then you have the right attitude. If you have given it a go and it's just not for you, create your own gay scene.

Do not rely on the internet as a window to the outside world. It can connect you with people all over the world, it's a powerful tool. Ensure you are responsible and take care with whom you speak to and exchange information with, do not give personal information, do not put yourself or anyone else at risk. There is nothing better than sending emails to one another, have a catch up on Skype or writing a few jokes on a friends FaceBook page but there are limits. If you find a friend on the internet that sounds as if you could really have a strong friendship and you are meeting for the first time do the following:-

- Take a friend along with you
- Meet in a public place so there are plenty of people around
- Don't commit to meet for the whole day on the first meeting

If you both agree to meet at 9:30am and decide to spend the day together and for some reason or another it doesn't go well, you can rely on your time limit to save you. You can say you'll spend the morning or the afternoon together, meet for a coffee or a drink in a bar after work. If you both want to pursue a friendship or even a relationship then it will make it more enjoyable the next time you meet. If it doesn't go so well then you have lost nothing and you have remained safe in the process.

ALLY BAKER'S STORY

"I suppose I didn't really know I was gay until I was twenty. I know people say that they always knew I was (my dad being one of those people), which is great for them, but it didn't hit home with me until I reached my twenties I guess I had the odd crush or two on guys at school, but I didn't think much of it.   I still fancied girls and had girlfriends (my last one at age twenty), and I hadn't even met a gay guy until I went to university at the age of eighteen. Then let's just say I was "experimental" and enjoyed it. Then I had the stereotypical bi-sexual intermittent phase, before admitting I was gay to myself in my second year at university.

I was never bullied for being gay and for that I'm very lucky. Oddly enough school peers used to pick on me for being gay, even though at that time I wasn't - so it made the whole experience rather frustrating since I knew it not to be true. I'm not sure whether in most cases they meant it, or were just being your typical childish teenager.

Coming out was nerve-wracking, in a word. To be honest, I can't remember whether I told my university friends first, or my family. It was more than likely to be the latter, but I did it in a successive motion - simply one after the other. Once it was out, I had to tell everyone I cared about and those who cared about me.

My coming out was different from person to person. However, for the widest perspective, I'll describe how I approached it with my immediate family members. The first person I told was my older sister, Liz. She and I have always been close, especially from our later teens, and out of my three sisters, I thought she would be the most open to the idea (I was aware that she had a couple of gay friends already). I remember telling her in the kitchen of our old home - she had popped over to the house at lunchtime, and it was just the two of us. When I told her she smiled and hugged me, saying that I should have known she "would be alright with it". We discussed telling Dad, which Liz was quite nervous about. My father has always been a "man's man", he used to serve in the army, then became a fire-fighter and attended a working man's club; so she wasn't sure how he'd take it.

The next person I told was Mum. She had picked me up from the train station after my return from performing up at the Edinburgh Fringe Festival for two weeks that summer, and the whole journey home I was mulling over how to broach the subject. We had to stop at the traffic lights conveniently outside our house and I thought to myself that "if she takes the news badly and kicks me out the car, at least I'm not far away from home!" Then I blurted it out, and the first thing she said was "promise me you won't become promiscuous". Considering the thoughts I had running around my head, that hadn't factored into any of them, so it was a pretty funny moment! It was more of an automatic response rather than anything properly thought through, she later explained. Finally, I had to tell my dad. I'm not the closest to him, but still thought it important I tell him. We had arranged to go for a catch-up meal together, and I knew that his partner would be attending as well which was perfect – again. I though that if Dad kicked off at least he wouldn't lash out too badly in front of her. I think she had an inkling that I wanted to tell Dad something, as all the way through the meal she was asking about my friends, and if I was seeing someone. I guess this was an easy way to approach the topic, so I told Dad about my feelings. Surprisingly, he was absolutely fine about it as well, retorting that he'd always known, ever since I was five years old! I think I was more surprised by that statement.

I'd have to say that all my relationships with my friends and family have remained the same, so I have been very lucky. I often chat to Mum about guys and she's probably fed up of giving me so much advice. My sister is much the same, having visited me in Cardiff numerous times and gone gay clubbing with my friends and I. Last year she even came to Mardi Gras, after I'd raved about previous years' events. I'd have to say that coming out was the best thing I could have done - mainly to settle my own head more than anything. Before I did I became quite frustrated and snappish if anyone attempted to talk to me about my feelings, even though, as my friends, they could sense something was wrong. I suppose I had to wait until I was ready to accept it for myself before being able to discuss it. Before then it wouldn't have been real. This was helped by having so many understanding people around me.

I worked on the gay scene in Cardiff for about nine months, so I pretty much know the ins and outs. I certainly find it a fun, relaxed, welcoming (in general) and entertaining place to be. It can become quite draining though, and I've seen how people can allow it to overtake their lives - they live, breathe, and eat the scene, and everyday life seems to fade to the periphery. You also get the stereotypical cliques and bitchiness, but no great difference from the straight scene. I believe that, like with every scene, you have to find the comfortable balance between going out and taking a break - doing too much of either will not do you any favours in the long-run. I know some gay guys who prefer to remain anonymous to the gay scene, but I still enjoy it (though I tend to avoid all the politics), and most probably will for a while yet".

CHAPTER SIX

Head Over Heels For That Special Someone

Falling For Someone

Falling in love can be the best feeling in the world and it can be the worst too. The pain of relationships usually happens when you fall for the wrong person, falling for the right person but the relationship breaks down or you fall head over heels for the one person you can't have because they are straight or just because they are not attracted to you.

Ahhhhhhh, love is a wonderful thing and when it is done properly you smile without reason, you are full of the joys of spring even if we are in the bleak midwinter, everything just seems to look, feel, smell and taste better. This is known as the honeymoon period; it is actually the best part. It's the bit where you hide all your nasty habits – and this is the stage where bodily functions do not exists as you would not dream of breaking wind or burping in the company of your new love interest. We have all been there!

Love is probably the most powerful emotion of them all. Now for the science bit: Your emotions are a physiological and mental state which connects to your thoughts, feelings and behaviours. All these things are invisible; they are intangible however they can make us do crazy things which show themselves physically in our behaviour. When we are in love we experience feelings of guilt, jealousy, envy and pride so on occasions it can cloud our judgement and even our rational thinking.

Courtney Nydahl's Story

"It seems to me that I always liked girls even though I indentify with being bi-sexual, but it was something I knew I was supposed to hide and so I tried to focus on boys instead. I think I really knew who I was though, the first time I kissed a girl and felt that spark, and knew that I couldn't keep pretending.

I was never bullied for being bi-sexual. Very few people know that I am, and they understand that I keep it a secret for a reason. It is down to just telling those I trust and those I feel I want to tell instead of having to tell.

I tried to come out to my family many times over the last five years, but since everyone treated it as a joke or a 'funny little rebellion' I gave up on it, it just wasn't worth it. So I haven't told my immediate family, I suppose I could be considered as not being out, because coming out to my mom was a major failure. I tried talking to her, and then dropping hints, and then I just came out one day to her after her Bible study group. I suppose I snapped when they were talking about how "gays are appalling" which I called her on and she defended it by saying she was free to think that. Then I tried to explain to her that I liked girls and she laughed. So, it wasn't especially successful.

Doing it this way actually went better than I expected, aside from the fact that my mom is in total denial and I can't quite bring myself to try coming out to anyone else except my sister (who says she doesn't understand it, but that it's my choice) and my friend who is ridiculously supportive. It was a bit demeaning that she can't take me seriously enough to accept something that means so much to me. My relationship with my parents is now awkward, I suppose. My sister and I don't discuss it, and my mom doesn't refer to it unless I bring it up, and then it's me 'joking around and trying to embarrass her'. It couldn't be further from the truth. I feel better now I have got it off my chest; I just hope to have told my whole family by the end of the year.

When I was sixteen I dated a girl but it was just 'young love' – not that serious and I haven't dated much since then. There hasn't been much opportunity to be honest. I will meet the girl of my dreams one day; it is just a matter of time. I am happy and comfortable with myself. I am a good person, I live a respectable life and I believe that God hates haters more than he hates love".

Can Gaydar Be Fitted As An Optional Extra?

The word 'gaydar' is made up of the words gay and radar and it refers to the instinctive capability to gauge a person's sexual orientation as gay or bi-sexual. Non-verbal sensory information and perception are used such as mannerisms, social behaviours and stereotypes in order to establish a person's sexuality. Straight people can have a highly tuned gaydar too. There has been much speculation whether gaydar really exists. Are there such things as in-built devices that detect other gay folk? Some people have a very well tuned gaydar, some are state of the art and they can spot a gay person on the other side of the supermarket car park. As a gay person you will find it easier to notice other gay people through their behaviour, their mannerisms or by giving you the eye. Some people go undetected as they are more straight acting so they might get overlooked as they are not giving the indicators that shout 'Gay over here! Gay over here!' It can also be difficult to determine if someone is gay depending on how hard they are hiding their feelings, they may not have come out and they might not have some of the indicators you would normally associate with someone who is gay. For the record, I have met plenty of individuals both male and female who have had stereotypical characteristics that are associated with gay people and these people are 100 per cent heterosexual so be careful not to offend anyone, there is a lot to be said about judging books by their covers.

If you have not come out and you like someone who happens to be in a similar situation, the communication can ground to a halt on the basis that you are both hiding yourselves, you are not showing your true colours. This makes the job of finding a girlfriend or boyfriend quite difficult.

As you begin to socialise more you may find someone you like who is gay, don't get hung up on whether they fancy you or not, or if you fancy them. Take it easy, there will be obvious signals if they like you and you will not be able to hide the feelings you have for them, it is just natural and will happen without having to be forced. Take it how it comes and relax, it should be fun and exciting, not an obstacle course. Remember the following six things and you will not go far wrong.

- Be yourself. You already know the importance of being yourself, we have discussed that. Putting on an act is exhausting and if all goes well and they fall for you, they will undoubtedly be in love with the act instead of you - meaning they don't truly love you. It's not their fault; after all it is you that put on the act in the first place. Be yourself, you are better than any act.

- If you are unsure if someone is gay and you are fairly certain that they are gay, you could ask them. Think before you do this, they may become defensive as they have had to hide their sexuality just like you. Imagine if someone had asked you before coming out. You would have come back with a resounding 'No'!

- If you have found someone you like and they like you then enjoy your time together. Don't rush anything, go to the cinema, go to a music concert, go for a meal – do something you both enjoy.

- One thing that can work well if you truly like someone is to become friends first. By truly liking someone you will not care whether they will be interested in you or not, you just want to have them in your life just because it will make your world a better place. You will have people in your life already that enrich your world, one more would be fantastic and if something happens later on down the line, even better. Take care to control your eagerness, do not come across too keen as you do not want to be taken advantage of. There are some who will use your affection for their own gain, keep your wits about you.

- Refrain from being disillusioned if the person you have feelings for does not feel the same or is not gay. If you really like them then you can remain friends. The one thing you cannot do when it comes to relationships is force people to like or love you in return. There is someone out there for everyone, they usually come along when you least expect it.

- This is a little tip for the gay men. As a gay man, if you have acquired a close friend who happens to be female and you find yourself attracted to another guy when you're out and you think they like you too, send her over to make the introductions. This can work, I have been out and been approached by 'the female friend', as I was not available I had to decline but I did admire the young man for his good taste and his enterprise.

Handling Rejection

Rejection is something we all dread in our personal and professional lives, and it can cause great upset when it happens. The fear of rejection can hinder asking someone out or avoid a close relationship with another, it is important to address these fears whether it is you or you can see it in others.

As small children we do not want to hear the word 'no', if we have asked for something there is only one answer we want, and if we hear anything different then we throw ourselves on the floor kicking and screaming until we get our own way. Not the right attitude to have you'll agree but kids will be kids. This behaviour cannot be replicated in adulthood, there are times when you will hear 'no' or you might not get what you really want.

Many people are fearful of rejection; it is a very sensitive subject as many people find it a difficult topic to discuss, the best way to overcome the fear of rejection is by changing your state of mind. You will get what your mind focuses on, so only think of positive things, there have been many terms to describe this and the one that everyone has heard of is 'positive mental attitude' or PMA for short.

If you are in a relationship and you fear each day that you will be rejected then you are increasing the chance that this will happen and eventually it will. This fear can be responsible for you failing before you have even started, you want to approach that person you really like and ask them out, with your mind telling you 'they are going to say no, they are going to say no' then the likelihood is they will.

Say you are in a bar, you see someone you like, and you go over and ask them out. You are saying the right things but your body and mind are saying something completely different, you are not congruent with what you are asking, this will only lead to the other person declining your invitation. Change your mental state, imagine them saying *yes* and the feelings you have inside after they have said yes will give you the confidence you need to go over there and get them. You do not have to be arrogant or too self assured, be yourself, a confident and positive you.

If they say yes then it is the most fantastic feeling in the world, you can begin your friendship and enjoy all the things that come with new romance, if the answer is 'no', it is not the end of the world. It is not 'no' to you, it is just *no* to the situation.

JASON HERNANDEZ'S STORY

"I realised I was gay a little later in life than most. It was when I fell in love with another man, at the age of thirty-three. Only in hindsight could I see I should have known sooner.

I was never bullied for being gay, any bullying I was subjected to was for being a shy, sensitive boy, not interested in typically "boyish" things (and I was small for my age). Some of that may have been the result of being gay, but I was not explicitly known to be gay then.

My coming out can only be described as painful, since I came out first to the man I loved, and he was not interested. Word got around the
84

division (I was in the Navy at the time), and I had the added worry the upper chain of command would find out. But coming out to my parents was a relief - they still love me the same as ever.

The whole thing went horribly wrong in that I never did get into a relationship with the guy, and my heart got fixated on him for two years afterward, until he had to cut off our friendship. When it came to my family it went better than I thought, as they treated me with love and respect and they took it in their stride. I am aware that I am unusually lucky to have had such understanding parents; many go through turmoil because they have to deal with the additional pressure from the parents.

I say that coming out is just part of living a genuine life, which everyone needs to do if they want to love the person in the mirror.

My first relationship happened about a year-and-a-half after coming out. It was with a man I met at Church. He initiated the relationship, and I went with it because I was still sad over the one I didn't get. He was the kindest man I have ever known, and we still have phone conversations - we never actually broke up, just both moved away and couldn't see each other anymore.

When it comes to religion I have come to a different point in my faith now, and not just because I am gay. There are a whole lot of traditional teachings of my faith that just don't seem to square with the real world. I have in many ways had to blaze my own trail - which is fitting, since I never was one to appreciate being told what to do or think anyway. Honestly, there are times when I wonder if fundamentalist Christianity is the apostate church of Revelation; it seems to have so little of Jesus in it, despite all the constant use of His Name. Lately I'm coming around more to Cosmic Christ theology, a la Matthew Fox.

I have only one thing to say when it comes to the gay scene: if you want to find Mr. Right, you're not going to find him by sleeping around. To find quality, you have to be quality; to get with Mr. Right; you need to be the kind of person Mr. Right would actually want. You can be either "the lady or the tramp"; your choice will affect who you end up with.

The one thing I have never been able to get my head around is the whole issue of gender. Take me for example, I am considered reasonably "well endowed", judging by peoples reactions to my penis when they see it, but honestly, I don't really like it. It gets in the way of wearing the kind of clothes I like, and I have actually considered a reduction. Just you try to find any information on the Internet about penis reductions! Everyone so worships the god of "bigger is better", the only references you find to reductions are sarcastic, as if you can't possibly be serious. However I am serious. All my life, I have wished I could have been genderless, neither male nor female, so as to avoid all the foolish gender-based expectations in society. I've heard of sexual reassignment surgery; is there such a thing as sex removal surgery?"

The Shoe Being On The Other Foot

You know the importance of treating others as you would like to be treated, should you find yourself in a position where you have to reject someone for whatever reason, speak to them with respect in a way that you would want to be spoken to. You do not have to explain yourself just give them a genuine and honest answer, 'I am sorry but I am not looking to get into a relationship right now' is far easier for the recipient to hear rather than 'Sorry but you just don't do it for me'. What goes around will come around remember, good or bad.

CHAPTER SEVEN

Dealing With Relationships, Break Ups And Mother Nature

Relationships and all the things that go with them are a never ending topic of infinite aspects. If anyone could create a formula or potion that created the perfect relationship then we would not need Life Coaches, Counsellors and all those other professionals who pick up the pieces when relationships end.

The misconception that many people have is that relationships are all about sex. There is some truth in this. Many think that if the sex is wavering in quality or irregularity then there is no hope for the relationship. People never actually question why the sex is 'no good'; it is in fact the relationship that is no good. Everything in the relationship might be great and the only let down is the sex. It is most probably due to the fact this is the area where the connection is weak.

It is crucial that a long lasting relationship is built on friendship to begin with. This is done by dating and taking things slowly. This creates an excitement which turns into anticipation that keeps the flames of eagerness alight until you next see them. Friendship will always outlast love: This is a fact. If you think about the genuine, true friends you have and think about the people you have 'loved' over the years, it speaks for itself. It is important to establish a friendship with your partner as well as being lovers and do not be too hasty to say 'I Love You' because once those eternal words are said you can never take them back.

When I met Andrew in 2001, I was not looking for him; in fact I did not want to meet anyone. We spent the first three years just getting to know each other as individuals. We were exclusively dating and it was fun and exciting. It was even a little scary, enjoy it and don't rush it, I say this because you may have actually met the person you are going to grow old with. We based our relationship on the fact we were best friends and I would say that this is probably the best advice I can give. Before we met I had never had any previous relationships and he was the same. It was hugely difficult to know what to do, and there were no other books out there that helped with coming out or how to deal with the emotions of getting involved in your first proper gay relationship. I acknowledge that our relationship was unusual, and am aware at this point that our situation was unique.

Be Different

Many people have remarked on our relationship, we are a monogamous gay couple who have been committed to one another for the length of time that we have been together. We are proud of our relationship, the course of true love does not run smoothly, you deal with the rubbish life throws at you and it is far easier when there are two of you fighting the battle rather than being alone.

I guess what I'm saying is, do what your head and heart say. Give each of them equal chance to voice what they feel and do what is right for you. Choosing a new partner is *not* the same as choosing a new car: Partners do not come with a log book giving you a full service history. So it is hugely important to get to know them and accept their 'faults' and enjoy exploring their good qualities.

The Secret Formula

The only formula to a winning relationship consists of common sense. This formula is transferrable to any type of relationship as the principals are the same. There may be one or two differences however it all begins with the three 'C's' which are communication, compassion and compromise.

COMMUNICATION

You have probably been told all too often to communicate, whether at school or at work. It is hugely important to demonstrate high levels of communication as no-one will ever know what you are thinking. You might be thinking that you have mastered this as you know how to speak and use body language. All too often relationships will go through periods of misunderstandings, purely down to a lack of communication. The easiest way to eradicate this is by telling your partner how you are feeling, remain calm and collected, as shouting and yelling will stop any useful communication. Discussion is the best form of approach to an issue and it is important that you talk as soon as you can – don't lose sight of what the discussion is about. Otherwise you may let it fester until you both decide to have a massive quarrel when it will all come out, usually in the wrong way and magnified. Had you decided to talk it through this could have been avoided. Do not keep your feelings to yourself, the best thing about having a partner is that a problem shared is a problem halved, once you have talked it through. Ignorance is only bliss because it is easier than facing up to the reality. The reality, however, is that keeping things to yourself will drive a wedge between you. So just say how you feel tactfully, ensuring you are taking your partners feelings into consideration. This moves us nicely onto compassion.

COMPASSION

I would say, as a general rule of thumb, never go to bed on an argument. It isn't helpful to be the one who says 'I told you so' and never wait for the other person to apologise if you are in the wrong. One thing to get used to when in a relationship is being compassionate if your partner is having a rotten time. They might be having problems at work, family issues or just a bit disenchanted with life. Your support will see them through this – this is quite a responsibility. Listen to them when they need to talk and give them words of wisdom when you feel they need to hear them, plenty of cuddles never go amiss either (if that's what they like). You may even face terrible life changing situations that will immediately affect you both, such as family bereavement. At times like this it is natural to want to run; in fact this is when we need to stay.

Remember, there are three sides to every story. There will be your side, your partner's side and there's the truth – which is usually a mixture of both. There is no point arguing over things; with a little communication and a bit of compassion it can be sorted out. Some people find it hugely difficult to compromise, just be your own person and do what you want to do and your partner can enjoy what they like to do – this way neither one is unhappy.

Let's say one person likes football and the other doesn't. Is it fair that the one who dislikes football has to endure a whole game of football for the love of the other partner? If you are the football lover and you are answering 'yes' then shame on you! If your significant other wants to watch football then arrange to catch up on things you have always been meaning to do. Meet that friend you promised to go shopping with and never got around to doing it. By letting your partner do what they want you will be able to do the things you enjoy that they don't. Plus when you go away and do something different you both have something to talk about later. It allows you to have space of your own.

It's all about creating the right balance and if you feel that in order to keep that balance you have to say "no" sometimes, then do it. Do not be the one who is running around trying to please the other, if you are afraid of losing your partner, this fear will cause exhaustion. You will become the weaker and less confident of the two, then it is no longer a partnership, it becomes a power trip.

TRUST

Trust is a must. There are couples in the world right now who have no trust when it comes to their significant other. There are those who check their partner's mobile phone, fit a tracker to the car to check their movements, or record their mileage to check it matches with the distance of their movements that day. You might think that these things are a little far fetched nevertheless this does happen. Think of the energy it takes to monitor all this activity, not to mention the emotional and mental strain through not really knowing. Any relationship that is built without trust will either fail dismally or will make your life a living nightmare.

If your partner is giving you cause to feel jealous or wary about their commitment to you, talk to them. If there is no trust then work out how you can build the trust because once trust is in place you can enjoy life, make the most of your time, put your energy into more important things. Trust gives you such a great feeling inside. Remember, you are in a relationship out of choice – it's not a prison sentence or fixed penalty. If it feels this way then get out now before anyone gets hurt.

RESPECT

It is not required to dwell on this subject for too long. The amount of couples who are in relationships at this moment where there is no respect may surprise you. Respect cannot be bought or demanded it is earned through communication, compassion, compromise and trust. I am sure you were brought up to respect your elders and those in authority. Respect is a two way thing, it must be earned, not created through position, power or birth right. Treat others like you wish to be treated yourself – if you are not receiving the respect you deserve from your partner then tackle it or be prepared to walk away.

ROMANCE

When you have been with a partner for a period of time you get fooled into believing that romance only comes around every Valentine's Day. When you first get together it is normal to want to be together all of the time, and when you are not together there will be texts, phone calls, emails and plenty of wall writing going on through social networking sites. It's hard to be without that person, though time away is vital to keep the excitement alive. Romance can do funny things to a person, like cancelling plans and arrangements made with friends or family just to be with the one you love. Sound familiar?

Enjoy these moments, it's easy to believe that they will last forever – and they can. On the other hand life takes its toll and changes happen that take these precious moments away. As the relationship becomes more serious and you decide to move in together you may miss those moments. They haven't gone; you are just in a different stage of the relationship. Don't drop friends just because you have a new partner, go out with friends for an evening as the time apart will make the heart grow fonder. Do not take your relationship for granted, appreciate that the same spark is still there it's just not so apparent now because you see the love of your life everyday.

Why should dates stop just because there is a house and a mortgage involved? Keep going on dates with one another. Decide on one evening a week that would be suitable to go out together, it could be just as a couple, or as a group of friends, or with other couples. Monday evening is a great night for doing this as this can be your reward for getting through the first day of the working week and it eases you in gently for the week ahead. Or it could be a Friday night which can be a celebration of the start of the weekend. Just have fun and put that day in your diary!

Leave The Past In The Past

Apart from gay people hiding in the closet we have also had a bad habit of putting our skeletons in there too, and after a while it becomes a necessity to spring clean. We all have a past and many of us like to leave the bad things hidden so that we hope that it never gets discovered and this can have a real impact on how we behave and feel at this point in time. It is highly unlikely that you or your current or future partner hasn't had any previous relationships. When the relationship comes to an end, you suddenly have a past and then go on to measure other future partners on the mistakes of the past, more often than not. If a past relationship has left feelings of hurt, deception and betrayal it is not set in stone that this will happen again. Perhaps you or your partner has had many previous relationships and this has left questions about commitment. It is a fair point and if any relationship is going to get off the ground then it needs to start afresh. Do not use past performances as a measure of the things that are still to come. Keep an open and positive mind and who knows what amazing things will blossom. The past is just history... or herstory.

Gay Marriage

So, things have been going well and you both have decided that you want to commit to one another fully and celebrate your love in front of your family and friends. Sure, straight couples have celebrated the union in marriage so why should gay people be any different.

Gay Marriages are only permitted and recognised in exactly the same way as a heterosexual marriage in: Belgium, Canada, Netherlands, Norway, South Africa, Spain and Sweden.

In much of Europe, 'Civil Partnerships' or 'Unions' exist which give similar rights to gay couples. In the United Kingdom these were brought in to effect in December 2005.

Despite the massive publicity gay marriage has drawn over the last few years, it is interesting to note that at present same sex marriage is permitted in only five of the fifty states of the United States of America. New York for example recognises gay marriages performed elsewhere for the purpose of state laws including divorce, but does not permit gay weddings to take place. Although much of the population of the USA seem tolerant of gay culture, public votes in more than 30 states have voted against allowing gay couples to become legally married.

Many other countries around the world have not made any provision to recognise the rights of gay married couples.

GARETH LLOYD-RICHARDS' STORY

"I think I knew I was different from a very early age but it took a few years to realise that I preferred boys to girls, despite this I still felt the need to date girls until the age of sixteen as it was what all the other boys were doing.

I decided that sixth form was the time to come out as being gay. I first came out to my closest friends who were shocked at the time, but happy that I chose to tell them. Even my ex girlfriends at the time remain close friends until this day. Although my friends were okay, I did experience some problems with other people in my school but they were in the minority so it didn't affect me much and I had a lot of support from my friends.

For the next couple of years it was great, I had the confidence to visit my local gay clubs as I now had friends who could come with me. From visiting clubs on the gay scene I soon realised that there was quite a large group of gay and lesbians in my area and as a result I made a lot of close friends. Despite living in the South Wales Valleys I never really had any serious problems with the fact I was gay. A few comments and names were called but nothing too serious; in a way I think I was very lucky compared to other people in the same situation.

When I reached eighteen I decided it was time to tell my close family, obviously I was very nervous and decided to tackle the most difficult person head on, my father. He was very supportive and understanding which caught me by surprise as I was expecting a rough time. Then I told my mother who took some time to get used to it, she worried about the problems I may have in the future by being gay but after a while she came to accept it and is happy for me.

Both my younger sisters were not surprised at all as they both had suspected it early on, gradually it spread throughout my family and after a year or so it became the norm. My biggest disappointment is the fact that I am unable to tell my great grandfather despite us being so close, he is very elderly and from that generation who would be very disapproving of my lifestyle and find it hard to understand.

Looking back I think I had an easy ride, and it was the best thing I have ever done. Three years ago I met my partner Jonathan and we married in August 2009. Both our families and friends were very happy and supportive towards us and we have now settled into married life. We felt that time had come to show the world our commitment to one another and we were proud to be together".

94

Dealing With Break Ups?

Dealing with a break up is a dreadful process and it very rarely goes smoothly. It is necessary; it can be an emotional drain to stay in a relationship that no longer fulfils. Remaining in an unhappy relationship that fills you with dread is not at all healthy for you. Ending a relationship may mean you are free, yet there is a need to deal with the sadness it brings and it is crucial to adjust as your relationship status reverts back to single.

WHERE DID IT ALL GO WRONG?

It is always easy to blame yourself if you have no control over the relationship break up, and it's also very easy to blame the other person. It is extremely difficult when a long term relationship ends. The amount of time invested in the relationship can seem like wasted time and it is soul destroying when the relationship slowly starts unravelling at the seams. This is usually a slow process where neither one actually sees the end coming, it leads to both parties feeling uneasy and discontented before coming to the conclusion it is over.

It can also come to an end more abruptly where one partner becomes unfulfilled and the other is blissfully ignorant of the other's unhappiness. In most cases the dissatisfied partner might end the relationship after finding someone else.

The break up can lead to obsessing about where it all went wrong and then analysing each detail and apportioning blame, which will not help. It is easy to re-run all the arguments and disagreements to see where it all went wrong – you can drive yourself crazy doing this. If the break up is obvious, learn from it and move on. It may sound cold and heartless; as experience of losing that special person from your life brings a lot of heartache. However accepting this is crucial. This will shape your future relationships.

If the break up happens and the reason is not so obvious; then delve a little deeper – meet with your partner and find out what caused the break up. It may answer some questions that will help you both move on. You might feel better knowing the real reasons instead of being suspended in limbo and they might feel better having got a few things off their chest, even in these circumstances communication is still the best policy. And I guess they call this *closure*.

If the break up is still raw and you both need time apart to re-adjust then arrange a meeting when things have settled down, then the hatchet can be well and truly buried – preferably not in the other person's back. Do not rake up the past, begin throwing insults or apportioning blame it will not benefit the situation. Take the lessons from these circumstances in order to grow; making the decision to move forward might help a friendship to blossom.

IT WILL NEVER BE THE RIGHT TIME

Coming to the conclusion that you are going to end your relationship with your partner is a big decision; you will be looking for excuses to hold off telling them how you really feel. That's natural. Do not stay in the relationship just for the sake of your partner; it is not fair on you and it is certainly not fair on them. It will be easy to find a multitude of excuses to postpone telling them. 'I'll tell them when they are stronger', 'When I have saved enough money' or 'I'll do it after Christmas'. If you are absolutely sure that the relationship must end then you need to ask for help from friends and family to help with accommodation, perhaps borrow some money and support your brave decision.

Take a little care in how you tell your partner that the relationship is coming to an end, show them respect and be tactful. It is amazing how many people prefer to take their partners on national television to break up or announce an indiscretion, rather than sitting them down and telling them one to one without the humiliation of being told in front of millions of viewers.

It is vitally important to be honest and not hurt the other person's feelings. If the relationship you are ending is relatively new and you want to end it perhaps it might be kinder to give them a generalisation rather than a list as to why the relationship is ending – it's less brutal. If
96

you are ending a long term relationship this needs to be discussed calmly and quietly. The truth is highly important, there may be questions from both ends, and they will need to be answered in order to move on.

Relationships end every day for many different reasons. Show yourself and your partner respect, do it face to face. As a word of advice it is not the best idea to break up with someone via:

- Telephone
- Email
- Text message
- Note pinned to the fridge door

Relationships have ended this way in the past for others. It is neither kind nor respectful - do it properly.

MOURNING THE LOSS

Leaving a relationship that was once fun, exciting and fulfilling can be a massive blow, it is normal to feel pangs of loneliness, even regret and only time will heal the loss. There is no cheating these feelings it will take time to get over the loss, like any grieving. Many have likened these feelings to those experienced during mourning; it is very similar to the grieving process that occurs when we have lost a loved one through death. They are expected to still walk through the door at a certain time, be brought to mind when a song plays on the radio or when you catch the sudden whiff of a scent they used to wear. Without them you will have to go to bed alone and wake alone; you will leave for work and return to an empty house. Give yourself time to get over them and work through it. Do not use the classic re-bound state and allow yourself to get caught up in another relationship just because you need comfort and company – it really will be out of the frying pan and into the fire. It's all too easy.

Enjoy time alone, get to know yourself again and be comfortable with your own company. You will know when the time is right to find that someone special. Rushing into another relationship without careful consideration will only result in another failure. Time it well and abstain from leaving it so long you have lost the confidence and drive to get back out there.

MOVING FORWARD

Daunting as it is to think about life after a break up, it will take time to move forward and look to a brighter future. Use those around to pull you through, rely on those nearest and dearest who can help in the rebuilding of confidence, self-esteem and a positive outlook. Remember, calling him or her isn't a great idea – let things be, you will only regret it if you do.

There's no dignity in a drunken phone call.

Take some time out from being in the relationship and consider the following as this can help.

- Love Yourself – It has never been a more perfect time to take a holiday, either alone, with a close friend or as a group of friends. Buy a few new clothes, book a holiday that is within your budget and get out there to re-charge your batteries. If you'd prefer you could stay in and sing along to the Bridget Jones movie on DVD.

- Spring Clean – Start afresh by clearing out all the reminders of what once was. Box your partners CD and DVD collections, put their possessions that have been left at your place in a box and return them. It is a fresh start; it is out with the old and in with the new you. This process will help you move forward.

- Clear Out – When you have cleared the memories from the house, you need to clear out too. Do not mope around the house. You are still the same you, do the things you enjoy, get the gang together for a great night out or in.

- Catch Up – Do you remember what it was like to meet your friends for coffee, go shopping on a whim or cook a meal on a Friday night for the latest gossip from your pals? If so, think how much fun you are going to have reminding yourself again. Get your phone book out, get the piggy bank out and get that cook book from under the shorter leg of the dining table.

Little Voice

We all have an inner voice in our head, you know the one that says "Don't rest that plate there, it will fall". Then we ignore it and then what happens, we say "I should have listened". Well, sometimes we have to be selective and decide not to listen to some of the inner voices. By the way these inner voices are nothing to worry about; you are not losing your mind. It is just the thoughts in your head playing out, they often put us down when we do something wrong. We all have an inner voice, but some people's inner voice might put them down and tell them that they are hopeless. In most cases it is in fact their voice. This is one of the techniques I discovered when studying for my NLP (Neuro-Linguistic Programming) Practitioner qualification. NLP is like software for the mind, you can re-programme your thoughts so you can safely change your association to a particular inner voice, memory or event.

This is how you can banish them, or at least change them so they sing to your tune. This will work by the way if you have hurtful things in your head that may remind you of your partner. It might be something hurtful they said or just something you need to break the association in order to move forward.

For the purpose of this exercise we will call the inner voice, little voice. You see by the end, no matter what the circumstances, you can modify this to suit the voice you are looking to change.

1. Listen to the little voice. There might be more than one, but let's do this one at a time. Where is it coming from...? Your

head, if so where, what part or can you hear it near your ear... which side?

2. Is it a voice you recognise, is it your voice or that of someone you know? Do you like the tone of it, does it sound casual and friendly, or is it aggressive and hostile?

3. Now you are concentrating on the little voice, how do you feel? Take a few moments and listen, think how you feel... really feel it.

4. Now let the voice travel to an insignificant part of the body. Out of the mind and into your thumb or one of your toes. Does that change the impact it has on you? It can't speak in your mind it has been moved, it is stuck there.

5. Now play with the tone and sound of the little voice. If it is aggressive and hostile then change it so it speaks the same words but in a different accent. An accent that is native to another country outside of what you are used to. Make it sound silly if you like, perhaps in a way you find comical.

6. Now, suggest to the little voice that you will be more inclined to listen if it changes it's attitude. To speak positively and give advice on how to do things right instead of criticising after the mistake has been made. To speak with a bit of respect and be a little more supportive and be a voice that you will want to listen to as opposed to wanting to ignore it.

You might feel silly doing this but don't because this can change the way you speak to yourself and also shape the way your little voice speaks to you. To have a little voice that supports and offers encouragement will actually make you a better and happier person. What do you have to lose by trying it?

When you have both moved on you may become friends again, you may even decide to take it a step further and become bed buddies.

This is not recommended, casual sex is what it is – casual. There is history between you and old feelings might get dug up and then you are in for a rollercoaster ride of events. Whilst you might have an 'arrangement' – when new relationships emerge either for you or your 'bed buddy' – things get complicated. This is not fair on the innocent parties and it is not fair on you either. There will be heartache as a consequence of this, you deserve better than this and so does your future partner.

Social Networking Site Warning:

Many people find it hugely annoying when a status on FaceBook gets updated on a daily basis with comments that result in the friend gushing about how wonderful their girlfriend or boyfriend is. It can be very annoying for the friends who have to endure these. It is nice to update your status when your partner does something nice for you but daily updates saying how much you miss them, how wonderful they are and what a fabulous relationship you have usually spells the opposite in reality so you need to ask yourself who it is you're trying to convince – thou doth protest too much.

The same can be said when things are not going so well. One of my old classmates (who is straight) was recently going through a divorce, which is painful in itself especially as there were kids involved. Her daily status updates where aimed at her soon-to-be ex-husband and he wasn't even on her friends list. It must have been hard for her, but do distant friends, old school friends, acquaintances and work colleagues want to read these. Private message those you know will understand when things go wrong instead of subjecting everyone to the abuse you have for one person. It was far easier for me to press the *hide* button than to have to read these daily.

CHAPTER EIGHT

The Birds And The Bees

It is vital that this topic is discussed however this is not a sex help manual with fancy illustrated drawings of men with handle bar moustaches or ladies who resemble 1970's television icons. This is dealing with the facts of the matter, sex guide books are hugely overrated anyway, just enjoy it – why not make your own books? Can you imagine anything worse than trying to carry out a sexual position whilst holding the manual to check to see you look similar to the illustration or photograph? I mean instructions are all very well when erecting flat pack furniture but come on people just have fun, don't worry if your legs are out of alignment. There is nothing more off putting during the throws of passion than your partner running off to get the spirit level to make sure you are in complete alignment with the recommendations of the Karma Sutra. If this sounds like your partner, I might suggest that the next time you are at the library you get a few books on hypotenuse and Pythagoras then this will really work them up into an uncontrollable mess. You might even have the best time ever!

Right, now the ice breaker is done, lets get to the nitty gritty: Sex is Mother Nature's gift, something that can make a person feel wonderfully happy, empowered and just incredible when you do it with the right person. Whilst doing my research about how others see sex they say it is a good stress reliever and it burns calories too!

That aside as soppy as it sounds; there is the beauty of intimacy. It is sometimes forgotten how wonderful it is when two people who genuinely care for each other become one. The gay scene has been notoriously labelled as sleazy and that sex is just a function rather than an emotional connection. It can also have the opposite effect; it has the power to make you feel vulnerable, uncomfortable, dirty and cheap. What's the difference? Well, it probably has something to do with the reasons you are doing it and with whom you are doing it.

At the time of writing this I am watching an old re-run of a US talk show where the guests are confessing to being sex addicts. Now, I never knew that people this bad existed; these people would go to any means just to have sex whenever and with whomever they wanted just to satisfy the need for sex like drink or drugs. It is frightening that they likened this addiction to a drug addiction, how alarming is that? There are people who have such a hunger, and uncontrollable need for sex that they will go to any lengths to get it. Some were happy with their addiction, sleeping with countless people in order to feel empowered, adored and wanted. It took the final guest to say how it had ruined her life, but with the assistance of counselling she is now 'sex-clean'. I was sat there open mouthed thinking 'what, this woman isn't going to have sex ever again' but she simply meant that she is now in a loving and meaningful relationship where she is only with her partner and she no longer needs sex from a multitude of people to feel satisfied.

When you live the life of the single man or woman and you decide that you can only find fulfilment or a sense of self-worth by sleeping with countless people you will soon burn out and come crashing down with a huge bang. Only when you respect yourself, and then respect others will you become satisfied with your life and yourself, you will find sex to be something that enriches your life as opposed to something that can only make you happy. It is merely a component of a happy relationship.

The Right Time To Start Having Sex

When we open the glossy magazines, newspapers or switch on the television we are faced with sex. It feels like all the world is having sex and we can feel pressured by the media, by comparing ourselves to our friends or by our partner. You should only do it when you are ready; it needs to be for the right reasons and it is only you that knows what they are.

Do not be fooled into sex with pressure from your partner saying "If you loved me then you would do it" or 'I'll leave you if you can't do this one little thing for me'. Remember, it maybe a little thing to them but a big thing to you so if they want to leave, fine. Point to the door and tell them not to let it hit them in the backside on the way out. *Do not* be a door mat and do not be fooled into sex. The greatest thing you were ever given was the power of free will, you will know when it is right: Trust me. You will not know when until it happens but you will know.

The same must be said from the other side too, you might be ready for sex but your partner might not be, you wouldn't like to be pressured so make sure that they are ready.

This is not aimed solely at those who are contemplating losing their virginity either. You might not be a virgin but having just found a new partner you might want to take time to explore the friendship side first; you can explore the sexual side when you are both ready.

Can't Get Out Of Bed Syndrome

When you first become physically intimate with your partner it may become impossible to tear yourself away from the bed. All you want to do is have sex and plenty of it. It is new and exciting; this display of affection shows the other that they are attractive. As time goes on and you both become more comfortable with one another these urges tend to cool a little. It does not mean that you are no longer attracted to one another and it is time to move on to someone else, it's quite the opposite. It means that you have both grown closer and there is more between you than sex and you will establish your role within the relationship, by this I don't mean 'who is the man, and who is the woman' I am implying that you will get a bit of structure and routine which as organised individuals you will need in order to get a sense of security to feel part of the unit, the sex will remain enjoyable and relaxed.

Communication

'Sex is a naughty word and should never be spoken about and you should only do it with the lights off'. I am kidding of course; these are things you are bound to have heard over the years, I find it really amusing. No wonder the Victorians didn't smile, they were doing it all wrong. The communication that was mentioned earlier in Chapter

Seven must carry on to the bedroom, you have to talk about sex with your partner, it is not required that you put the kettle on and sit them down with a nice cup of tea. You do, however, need to talk about it as communication is the only way both you and your partner can grow together. There might be something you want to try in the bedroom and have not been sure how to bring it up. This is simple, just ask. If they are open to it then great, if it is not for them then let it remain a fantasy. Talking is vital, if your partner doesn't know what drives you crazy or turns you off how are they going to know to do it more or stop altogether? Talk to each other, life is too short for mind reading.

I have a theory about fantasies, when you have fulfilled it, it is no longer a fantasy so then you find another and another and another. Usually they get more and more extreme each time you fulfil the last. Be sure to give it plenty of thought if you want something to remain a fantasy or become a reality.

There is a difference between fantasies and being adventurous, it's your call.

The Legal Age

We all have an obligation to ourselves and others to make sure that we are acting sensibly and within the law. When sex is involved all rational thinking goes out of the window, people forget themselves and the importance of contraception and that little matter of the age of the other partner gets forgotten too. This maybe a little matter to some but it is hugely important that the other person is of legal age so take care and make sure you know about the person you are going to share a special moment with.

The legal age of consent varies from country to country and also the sexual orientation of the couples taking part. For example, sex between a man and a woman in England, Scotland and Wales is 16 years of age and in Northern Ireland, it is 17.

The legal age of consent for anal sex between a man and a woman in England and Wales is 18 years of age and the laws in Scotland say it is

16 years of age and it is illegal in Northern Ireland for a man and woman to engage in anal sex. In the UK the legal age of consent for anal sex between two men is 16 years of age.

There is no strict guideline or law on the age of consent between two women however certain laws have suggested that two women who engaged in consensual sex must be over 16 years of age in England, Wales and Scotland and in Northern Ireland the age is 17 years of age.

It's Your Virginity

There is no rush to get rid of your virginity, it doesn't take up any room and when you have given it away then it is gone for good, make sure that it is special. It is not recommended that you give it away on a drunken night out; I have known those who have given their virginity away and hardly remember a thing. It is up to you how you choose to, with whom you do it, whatever you decide; make sure it is a happy memory and not an unhappy or fuzzy nightmare. Because it will be one you remember, good or bad.

I have always been picky about my shoes, and they only go on my feet so when it come to losing my virginity I wanted to be with the person I was going to spend the rest of my life with. I met Andrew, I was not that keen on him and you will find out why in Chapter Seventeen. But I also knew that I was going to spend the rest of my life with him. My virginity was the biggest gift I had to give someone. It was all mine, I could keep it as long as I wanted or give it away whenever I wanted, to whomever I wanted. There was no pressure and it was wonderful and you get a tremendous feeling when, years later, you are still with the person who you have grown close to both physically and mentally. By saying this I am not taking the moral high ground, you do not need to be with the person who you gave your virginity to, relationships often don't work out, just go in with a clear mind of what is right for you at that time. Give your virginity away to someone you love, don't throw it away.

Brian Gold's Story

"I knew I was gay pretty much my whole life, when I was between the age of thirteen and fifteen years old I would try to sneak looks at Playboy and Penthouse magazine, especially once I realised that there were sometimes men in the photos. I'm embarrassed now that I ever even looked at naked women.

I was bullied for being gay way before coming out; from the time I started in Junior School and finished up in Grammar School. Kids can be cruel can't they? I was often called a "faggot" or "homo" and always felt alienated as never being part of the "in" crowd.

When I came out it was a traumatic time, at first. A lot of, well not self-loathing exactly, more like "It's fine for everyone else, but NOT for me" came about. It was easier than I thought it would be after a very short time of coming to terms with my sexuality. Acceptance by friends helped a lot, and the realisation that "I am what I am, and what I am needs no excuses" went a long way. I was very happy and proud of myself; it took guts to do it.

I slowly began telling my closest friends who were all very supportive. I only told my mom after I met someone who was quite special to me. She told me one day I'd make a great father. I told her I didn't intend to have children. She asked if it was because I didn't want any, or if it was "something else". moms ALWAYS know! It was a relief in many ways, no more pretending or having to live a lie.

I waited a few more years before telling my father. He and my partner at the time, Vince, already got along well. I figured that Dad just didn't want to know. So the day he asked me if he should invite Vince to his wedding when he remarried, I said yes and told him why. My dad was a Ph.D. and living in Greenwich Village. He said he was very surprised! Guess the only image he'd ever had of gay people were the most obvious ones, and drag queens of course. He even asked me at first if I thought I could change. I asked if he thought that he could change. From then until the end of his life last year, Vince was like a son to him. He is still like a son to my mother and my father's wife, Celine.

108

I thought it might go horribly wrong when I came out, but it didn't and I am happy with the result. I feel that if somebody has a problem with it, that it is their problem, not mine. I have always been happy to assist anyone who wants to get a better understanding of what it is to be gay if they want to know.

There is nobody in my life that is important to me who does not know that I'm gay. It's not an issue, just as it should be. I don't ask them about their heterosexuality and they don't ask me about my homosexuality. I feel free to talk about a boyfriend or a partner if I want to.

Coming out was neither the best thing nor the worst thing I have ever done but it was certainly the most honest, and in some cases, the most difficult. I have never suffered with my faith as I am not a religious person. I am everything a Christian should be; kind, generous, loving and caring but I do not practice religion. I do say however "Dear Lord, please save us from your followers".

I'm not and never have been into the gay scene. And to be very honest, I'm often pretty annoyed that everyone thinks that all homosexuals are "like that". Nobody speaks for me. Gays and lesbians are as diverse as the rest of humankind. Some like and enjoy the gay scene whilst others don't. Just don't think that we all do!

Then came the time of when I lost my virginity. I "messed around" (exploring the male form if you like) with someone shortly after I turned twenty-three. I was not at all attracted to this guy; we didn't go the whole way but just experimented. This was my first sexual experience. I felt filthy. I felt as though I had betrayed my own moral code. I'm not sure where that "code" came from. It certainly was NOT from my parents or family. I actually lost my virginity around six months later with a wonderful guy named Carlo. I was working as a flight attendant and had a week layover in Anchorage, Alaska. It was December, so there was not much daylight, and not much to do there either. Late one afternoon while sitting in the lobby, the crew of another airline arrived and was checking in. There was Carlo at the front desk, checking in while I was checking him out. He was gorgeous. I walked straight up to him and asked what airline he was with. I wondered if Carlo might have been gay and my suspicions were confirmed when he telephoned my room. We met up that evening and we shared an incredibly beautiful, romantic, and far too short a time together in Anchorage. He had to leave the next day. He made the mistake of saying those three dangerous words, "I love you". I actually had the right response; I laughed and said, "How can you say you love me? You don't even know me!". He said "I don't know how I know, I just know".

As I had plenty of time to think in uneventful Anchorage I had convinced myself that he must have really meant it, and that I loved him too. I was writing to him daily and couldn't wait to get home to all the cards and letters that he surely must have sent me. Of course, there were none when I got home.

The story with Carlo ends well though. We did see each other several times after that, and we called each other and wrote. He was always very sweet with me, and never hurt me at all. He explained that he really did love me, just not in the way that I had hoped. He let me down very easily. I have always been a hopeless romantic. I still believe that "having sex" is when you either don't know or barely know the person you're with. "Making love" is when you and the person you are with are expressing a physical manifestation of the love that you feel for each other.

Since then I have met Mr. Right several times; my longest relationship lasted almost seven years. My current relationship, of six years has been turbulent to put it mildly. At present New York doesn't allow civil unions. My partner is Guatemalan, lives in Guatemala, and has no US visa. I commute between Guatemala and New York – that is one hell of a long-distance relationship! I am a flight attendant so it does make it a bit easier, but it's still really tough on both of us.

I do not regret losing my virginity with Carlo, I felt wonderful, special and yes, even loved. Time passed and we fell out of touch for a while, but we are now once again in touch, and I visited him and his husband with my partner in Holland where they now reside. It was absolutely wonderful to see him again".

110

Open Relationships

The typical relationship between two people is usually monogamous, built on love, respect and trust. These are core values and it is what many pride themselves on having, it shows loyalty and exclusivity to that one person.

Open relationships or polyamorous relationships if you want to be technical about it, are very popular in gay culture because when you decide you are flying the open relationship banner, you can have your cake and eat it, and also have extra fruit, ice cream and anything that comes with it. There are those who find that monogamous relationships are not for them therefore they can experience sex outside their relationship. An open relationship, like a monogamous relationship, comes with rules as well. If both individuals are running around having sexual encounters with others behind their back then there is something very wrong with this relationship. There needs to be communication, perhaps both persons do not want to know all the details but at least sort out what is acceptable and what is not, this way you are sure to have a very successful open relationship. Communication is the key to a successful relationship.

It is also important as a word of caution to mention the need for protection to reduce the likelihood of STDs or other fatal illnesses.

Three's A Crowd

There are some couples who find that their relationship is hugely successful as a result of adding a third person to the mix. The third person might integrate into the relationship fully or just occasionally. Again this is only done when communication is used at its best. If you are one of those people who want to be in a monogamous relationship then settling down with someone who wants to be in an open relationship or adding a third person will only bring you heartache so make sure you understand what you both want. Again ground rules are crucial here, perhaps you will only engage in certain acts with the third person and there might be things that are off limits that are only to be done with you and your partner.

It is normal that once you commit to this then you might feel angry, sad or jealous as you come to the realisation that this is not for you. You should communicate this to your partner right away, and also show them the same understanding, so if you are fine with it and they are uncomfortable then pull the plug or risk ruining your relationship. You see a common theme running through here - *Communication*.

Keep in mind, you should feel no pressure and should not be pressured in to it, if at anytime you feel it is not right then speak up.

Casual Sex

When you have just come out and the unbearable weight has been lifted from your shoulders it is absolutely normal to explore your sexuality in all areas. When it comes to sex I have known many people who have hopped from one bed to another in order to find out what they like and what they don't like. It is as though they don't know what to choose so they have to sample a little of everything on the menu. This is known as casual sex and it is often referred to as a 'one night stand' and this is where you might find someone at a club, a bar or at any social or work gathering and you decide to have a sexual encounter. Casual sex can also be opened up to mean sex with a bed buddy or with a friend for occasional sex or just on a one-off basis.

I knew from the age when you start thinking about sex that I didn't want just casual sex, it is not for everybody, it wasn't for me, when I met Mr. Right then I decided that I wanted to be monogamous and remain in one relationship. It is difficult as there is a stereotype that all gay men or women want casual sex whenever and wherever they can get it, this is not true. There are those who want to find the right person the first time round. I do not condemn those who do want to explore their sexuality by having casual sex, it's down to personal choice as long as people play safe and I don't just mean using protection. You have to remember that there is also your personal safety to consider.

112

There are three ways to look after your personal safety when you are meeting someone for casual sex.

- Tell a friend where you are going, give them the other persons name, address and mobile number if you have it.

- If you don't have these details then arrange to call your friend with these details once you have gone to their home, so they know where you are and that you are safe.

- Arrange to meet your friend for a catch up the following day either at home or while you are out and about.

Casual sex is all very well as long as everyone involved is aware that it is just casual, if it becomes more than this then you are moving into a different territory and this is a well known place called 'Relationship'. I would love to be able to say that relationships make you blissfully happy and it can be compared to something out of a Disney animation but it's not. In fact relationships usually consist of the bits that Walt Disney decided not to include when he first created Snow White and The Seven Dwarfs. Many people have successful, balanced relationships where both are happy, but there are some who are very unhappy. Do not be one of the latter.

Social Networking Site Warning:

Promiscuity is down to the individual, many have said that it is difficult to find true love whilst out on the scene and the same has been said about websites such as Gaydar. It is far easier to meet people for a one off encounter or a few casual flings, but it is harder to meet the person of your dreams. If you feel the need to put pictures on these websites that leave absolutely nothing to the imagination then the viewer knows exactly what you are looking for. If you decide to meet people this way then take care and use common sense.

With the birth of FaceBook, MySpace and all other similar websites the past you once lived can have a habit of coming around again. Past relationships may come knocking in the shape of a 'friend request', and old feelings can be resurrected. This has broken up the relationship of many couples both gay and straight. When thinking back to the past with all the excitement and thrill that once was, it is important to remember that you have moved on for a reason. Think very carefully before you decide to make your past your new future.

CHAPTER NINE

Protection, Protection, Protection

WARNING: This chapter has not been written to scare you or discourage you from any type of physical intimacy. It has been written to educate you, so that when you do find the person you want to physically bond with, you will know what steps need to be taken.

The Facts

Medical statistics reveal that over 60% of women and over 40% of men who have had a sexually transmitted disease or STI for short, didn't show any symptoms at all. I don't know about you but that bloody terrifies me.

It can be worrying and unpleasant having a sexually transmitted infection or disease, there is no need for concern they are preventable so long as you use protection. If you choose not to protect yourself then you are opening yourself up to a greater risk of disease, some are treatable, and some are not. Some leave you with consequences and problems that impact on all aspects of your life and those around you. The choice is yours. I am not saying this to scare you; I am just simply bringing it home now so you can start as you mean to go on.

Unprotected sex means having penetrative sex without using a condom. There are both male and female condoms and they both work as effectively, to reduce the chances of contracting HIV or any of the following sexually transmitted diseases:

Bacterial Vaginosis ▪ Chlamydia ▪ Genital Herpes ▪ Genital Warts ▪ Gonorrhoea ▪ Hepatitis A ▪ Hepatitis B ▪ Hepatitis C ▪ HIV and AIDS ▪ Pubic Lice ▪ Scabies ▪ Syphilis ▪ Thrush ▪ Trichomonas Vaginalis ▪ Urethristis

It has been estimated that there are 20,000 people in the UK who are HIV positive but don't know they've got it.

The number of people being treated for Chlamydia has increased by 206% in the last decade and the number of people being treated for Syphilis has increased by 1,949% and these were mainly found in the high-risk groups such as gay men.

STIs are not caught from sleeping around; they are simply caught through unprotected sex. We have all heard the false myth about you can't get pregnant the first time you sleep with someone, well this is the same. If there is sex involved and there is no protection there is always the possibility you may contract a sexually transmitted disease.

What's The Worst That Can Happen?

The HIV virus is the most fatal of the STIs because there is no cure for it, it weakens the immune system and slowly breaks down the bodies ability to defend itself. People do not die because of HIV – they die of other illnesses such as pneumonia, liver diseases and lymphoma.

Gonorrhoea shows itself by producing a green puss or discharge from the penis and many STIs do not show any symptoms and can result in infertility, heart disease and damage to the nervous system.

The most common and easily curable STI is Chlamydia – often there are no symptoms so many do not know they have it, again without immediate treatment this STI can lead to infertility. It has been estimated that at least one in ten young people under the age of 25 may be infected with it. Often people don't know they have it as these infections don't always show symptoms, but an infection, if left untreated could leave you unable to have children.

Trisha Jennings' Story

"I am a bi-sexual female born in the UK and now living in France. In January, I decided to take a trip to see a medical professional at my local

Genito-Urinary Medicine (GUM) Clinic. I had left it too late in the day because by the time I arrived it had shut. I dreaded going, firstly it is a highly embarrassing experience, and it is a little unpleasant too. I knew I had to go; I had already left it a few weeks and I kept putting it off week after week. I had plucked up so much courage to go there only to be disappointed when it was shut. I had a feeling I had contracted a sexually transmitted infection and wanted to be sure. As they were closed I went back home and carried on with life. I was almost sure I had contracted something from a guy I had a one night stand with at New Year.

The first symptom was a sore-throat, I convinced myself it was a cold but it got increasingly worse. I went to my GP and asked for antibiotics, I had them before for a severe throat infection so I just played on that. I didn't tell my GP about my suspicions of having an STI. I even thought the antibiotics might even clear it up – deluded or what? It did ease the pain and it subsided, I thought I had bounced back and I even went on to have sex with several other people.

A few months had passed and I found myself back at my GP surgery because I had swelling on my joints, my elbows and knees swelled, I had palpitations, breathing difficulties and chest pains. I was a mess. Again not arousing my doctors suspicions of my STI (and by this point I had pushed it to the back of my mind) I was signed off with anxiety and depression. I was almost sure that this was not the case. A few months passed and the symptoms became more controlled and I also became quite used to feeling like death-warmed-up. Again I went to my GP as my joints had become unbearably stiff, which was similar to what arthritis sufferers might have but being twenty-nine I though it impossible. My GP then confirmed what I had suspected all along, I was having the symptoms of the STI that I had contracted.

I was booked in to see a Rheumatologist who diagnosed my condition as reactive arthritis; this is more commonly known as Reiter's syndrome which is untreatable. It is an illness that is brought on by Gonorrhoea or Chlamydia.   The sore throat was the first symptom of having Gonorrhoea but although I was suspicious, I chose to ignore it. I now have arthritis, heart problems, eye problems and long term problems that affect my bladder, spine and joints.

Having done some research, I have found out my local GUM Clinic has a four-week waiting list to be seen by a medical practitioner, and some clinics have even closed their books to new patients due to the overwhelming number of infected patients".

What To Do?

The simple advice is to get yourself checked out by your GP. Remember that everything is 100 per cent confidential, even if your family doctor is your family friend the only people that will find out are those you tell. Yes, you might feel embarrassed, but you will not be the first person to present this to your doctor and you certainly will not be the last. Things have moved a long way since the time when a urethral syringe was inserted through the penis to inject mercury into the bladder for STIs.

Check your genitals to make sure there are no sores or blistering; if you find any abnormalities then you may be infected. The quicker you get to the GP the quicker it will be sorted.

No Excuses

Condoms are available in a wide range of colours, flavours and even sizes so there is no excuse for your sexual partner saying that they do not fit. There are allergy-free condoms for those with latex allergies and even condoms that are vegan friendly, which are free from animal products. They have thought of everything.

Relax and enjoy it. Sex is very rarely as intense as it is portrayed in movies and television, it can be ungraceful and uncoordinated but it can be as enjoyably intense. Never lose your head, always make sure that protection is used.

Visit **www.VarietyCondoms.com** for a variety of condoms for the UK, the USA and in fact anywhere in the world. It doesn't matter whether you or your partner has allergies to latex or you are vegan or larger sized condoms are required, they have it all. Even toughened condoms that are designed for anal intercourse, they give the added protection whilst not diminishing the enjoyment. They offer a fast reliable service and package everything discreetly.

JAMIE HURLEY'S STORY

"I am thirty years old and single. I was contacted recently by an ex-partner who said that I should get checked out as he has recently attended his local GUM Clinic for a routine check up and he was told the devastating news that he had contracted HIV from a former lover. He said I should get checked out too because we had unprotected sex during our eleven months together. I went straight to my GP who arranged my HIV test, they handled it really sensitively due to the fact I was at my wits end. The news came back that I too had contracted HIV.

My whole world fell apart. I went through the stages of anger and denial, and I have come out the other end. I have questioned God with the typical question of "Why me!?" I am angry because I have never been promiscuous, I have only been intimate with those I have been in relationships with, I have never been keen on the whole 'one night stand' thing. I loved sex and had plenty of it, but only with those I was committed to.

I am now being monitored by the professionals at the GUM Clinic a few times a year and thankfully I am not on any medication, this is a good thing so I'm told as my health has not deteriorated.

I have told my parents and close friends and family and they have been really supportive – they try to understand but they cannot understand what I am going through. Unless you are living with HIV then you can't ever know what it is like. I cannot say I have suffered any discrimination as I have not told anyone at work. If I did then I am sure they will look at me with all the clichés of 'a gay person suffering with a gay disease'. I do live in fear of discrimination and prejudice; I do feel isolated and alone. I also fear the illnesses I will have to endure as my body weakens and shuts down. I can't think about it too long as it really depresses me and I am not giving up on life. I have a good job which I really enjoy and I intend living life to the full and I have developed a positive mental attitude about living with my condition.

As for my former partner, we support each other and we speak regularly. It is nice to know I can pick up the phone to someone who will not look at me as 'damaged goods', it's nice that I can have time out alone when I am not in the mood for talking. I have met others who are learning to live with HIV from the people I meet at the local GUM Clinic. Again it's nice that people understand what I am going through and I am sure it is the same thing for them too.

With regards to my love life, I do not know what the future holds. I have many dilemmas to face with this subject. If I do not tell a potential partner then I am not being honest which means that it will go nowhere. If I tell them then they will either run a mile or I am risking my secret getting out should the relationship end. The other people I have met at the GUM Clinic have active sex lives with their partners – they will never be able to have unprotected sex with them but they have not lost the intimacy.

It has also opened my eyes when I hear the stories of how the people I meet at the GUM Clinic have contracted HIV. Some contracted it through drug use and using dirty needles, some through one night stands (heterosexuals I might add), and one was a police officer who was infected in the line of duty. I am optimistic that I will meet the right person one day who will accept and love me and who can look past my illness.

I end by saying that sexual health advice needs to start at school. I do not mean that it has to be the condom and the banana situation, but some age appropriate advice mentioning the pitfalls of unprotected sex. We need to adapt to the world of today, steering away from the subject of 'Is homosexuality right or wrong' or 'Should sex be performed by those out of wedlock' but just appreciate that same sex relationships are highly common, as is sex before marriage. If people are going to do it, then at least do it safely".

Reassuring Your Safety

There may be condoms being sold that do not offer the protection that one might expect; they may be made from poor materials. Make sure that the box carries the European CE symbol, a recognised safety standard. Novelty condoms also do not offer any protection so look out for that CE symbol.

- Always follow the instructions on the information leaflet inside the box.
- Never re-use a condom - use a new one every time.
- Change the condom if it has been worn for a while.
- Never use two condoms together – this will not add extra protection in fact it will have the opposite effect – this means do not wear two male condoms or a female and a male condom.
- Check the expiry date - condoms don't last forever.

Free condoms are often available; you will find free condoms at the following organisations:

- Family Planning Clinics
- NHS sexual health (GUM) clinics.
- Gay pubs and clubs.

You can also buy condoms from the following retailers:

- Pharmacists and drug stores
- Supermarkets - with self-serve checkouts no-one will know
- Petrol stations
- Vending machines in public toilets – both men and women
- Online shops offer great deals and discreet postage and packaging such as **www.VarietyCondoms.com**.

When ordering online be sure to get them from an online store or legitimate dealer rather than people selling them on eBay. There are some who sell the real thing on eBay, just make sure to ask the right questions, and always check that they carry the CE symbol.

"I recently lost my son Jonathan as the result of AIDS at the age of thirty-eight. He was diagnosed by our family doctor as having HIV about twelve years ago and it progressed to AIDS five years ago.

The care he received from the medical professionals who dealt with him was brilliant, such lovely people and they truly are the 'unsung heroes' that make a difference to those living with the illness and the family who support them.

As we lived in a small remote town in England there was very little money in the pot to help Jonathan and others who suffered with the same illness, although it is a different story in the bigger cities. Jonathan worked a large amount of time in London and the treatment he received was second to none. His condition worsened quite rapidly, he wasn't as strong as some and the illness took its toll on his very being. He moved back to our rural village and at the end he passed away with pneumonia, he did fight but as soon as he was diagnosed he was defeated.

He contracted it through unprotected sex, a costly mistake which meant that he left this world and a loving family far too early. Living in a rural location the local hospices and hospitals knew very little of HIV and AIDS so were unequipped to deal with Jonathan's condition. He suffered a painful death which might have been avoided had he had the support and knowledge of those hospices and hospitals in London".

When To Stop Using Condoms?

There may come a time when you decide that you no longer wish to use condoms, perhaps you have been with your partner for a while and this is the person you are staying with. It would be safe to continue the use of condoms until:

- You are both sure that neither of you have a STI or STD. I would recommend that you may want to have a check-up at the Sexual Health Clinic first to have the all clear and then start as you mean to go on.

- You are both certain that one of you will not go and have unprotected sex with someone else. It is probably a good idea to continue using condoms if you are in an open relationship.

- You are both certain that neither of you will be sharing drug injecting equipment with anyone.

Protection During Sex

ANAL SEX

If you are not actually sure what anal sex is, it is when the penis enters the anus. It has always been thought that anal sex was something that only gay men did, but did you know that statistics show that anal sex is not exclusive to gays and is practiced by a significant number of heterosexual people.

The lining of the anus is very thin and can be easily damaged during sex. Using condoms and water-based lubricants, such as KY Jelly, will help protect the lining and also prevent contracting STIs. Be careful of other forms of lubrication, such as Vaseline which is an oil-based lubricant, as these can cause condoms to split as they weaken the material, as can over-energetic thrusting. You can now buy specially toughened condoms that are designed for anal intercourse; these offer more protection for added piece of mind. Again you can visit **www.VarietyCondoms.com** for these.

ORAL SEX

Oral sex is where the penis is sucked and licked (known as fellatio), and this also applies to the vagina (cunnilingus) or the anus. Those who are giving and receiving oral sex can contract STIs; it is practiced by men and women both straight and gay and by adults of all ages.

The types of infections that can be passed on through oral sex are Herpes Type 1 which can cause cold sores around the mouth and Type 2 which can cause genital sores. You may also be at risk from Gonorrhoea and Chlamydia, which can infect the throat of the person who is giving oral sex and Syphilis, can cause an infection on the tongue and lips. Also, be aware receiving oral sex from someone with a cold sore could result in Herpes if you are unlucky.

Hepatitis B is a virus that is present in sexual fluids and blood, and can be transmitted during oral sex in a similar way to HIV. Hepatitis C is usually only contained in blood and may only be transmitted if there is blood present during oral sex.

Wearing condoms during oral sex can dramatically reduce the risk of STI transmission; there are a variety of flavoured condoms available that assist in making oral sex enjoyable whilst remaining safe.

RIMMING

Rimming is another display of oral sex, again this is popular among straight and gay couples and it is oral sex around the anus. Hepatitis A is a virus that is contained in faeces. In order to reduce the chance of infection, good anal hygiene before and after sex is crucial and this means that good oral hygiene before and after sex is vital too. Take care when brushing your teeth before oral sex as this can cause bleeding, any sores or open wound are susceptible to contracting infections and diseases. Faeces does not normally carry HIV but it can carry Hepatitis A and a large range of other organisms.

It would probably be wise to use a barrier such as a dental dam to lower the chances of any infections from Hepatitis A and any other range of intestinal parasites.

FISTING

This is something that will not appeal to everyone, fisting involves inserting the whole hand, starting with the fingers and sometimes the forearm into the vagina or anus.

WARNING: I am not a doctor but even someone with a fraction of common sense can work out that by sticking something that has the thickness of a fist or forearm into an area as delicate as your vagina or anus is probably not the best of ideas.

I am not disrespecting anyone who enjoys this in order to feel they have a fulfilled sex life, but what I am saying is that it's vital to use lots of lubricant and ensure that the receptive partner is very relaxed. Only do this if you are absolutely comfortable with it, if you feel unsure or half-hearted about this then under no circumstances should you be the receiving partner to this.

I must stress that care must be taken by the inserting partner to ensure that there is no risk of any internal injury. It is unlikely that an STI can be transmitted through fisting but if the inserting partner has burns, cuts or broken skin on the hand or forearm then the risk of infection does increase. As already mentioned Hepatitis B and C can be passed on by blood as well as HIV. There are surgical gloves available from health centres these will give a little more added protection from transmission through burns, cuts and broken skin.

FINGERING

This is where the vagina or anus is stimulated using the fingers, it is not common to spread STIs this way; however as with fisting there are still risks. If the inserting partner has any burns, cuts or sores regardless how small, the risk of passing or catching HIV or other blood transmitted infections like Hepatitis B or C is heavily increased. Once again surgical gloves will give some added protection. If you both decide that gloves are not to be worn then make sure that the inserting partner's hands are clean and free from cuts and good hygiene is being practiced.

DIPPING

This is where the penis is just dipped in the vagina or anus. This is not classed as full penetration but there is a chance of passing or contracting STIs as HIV can be transmitted through pre-ejaculate or precum as it is also known. Shallow insertion of the penis carries risks if there are any injuries, however small, in the anus or vagina. Using a condom even when dipping can protect against HIV, Hepatitis B and C. There is also a risk of contracting Chlamydia, Genital Herpes and Syphilis unless protection is used.

URINE AND FAECES

During sex two consenting adults might partake in 'golden showers' or 'watersports' as it is often called. This is where one partner will urinate on the other. If the receptive partner has no cuts or broken skin it carries a low risk of passing on any infection.

Again two consenting adults might take part in scat or poo play. Faeces, poo or excrement, call it what you will, contains organisms which can cause infection and illness eg e.coli. Faeces does not normally contain HIV, however it can contain Hepatitis A. There is a high chance of infection if the receptive partner has cuts or broken skin and also if the faeces comes into contact with the receptive partner's eyes or mouth.

This chapter is not offering sex education to you although it is only correct to raise awareness of the dangers that unprotected sex can cause. I don't have to tell you that sex is a natural desire, it is enjoyable, it is fun and you need to be aware of any risks. When you are presented with the facts you can enjoy a healthy and safe sex life and know that you are doing everything within your power to protect yourself and your partner.

I would like to thank the Sexual Health Line for their assistance. They do a fantastic job of raising awareness of the importance of sexual health. For those in the UK you can call them free (from the UK) on 0800 567 123 for help and advice regarding anything in this chapter or visit their website **www.CondomEssentialWear.co.uk**.

CHAPTER TEN

"... I Now Pronounce You Husband And Wife"

Let's look at men and women who have for a long time battled with their sexuality, the same way most people do when they realise they are attracted to the same sex. However their lives haven't exactly mapped out in the way they might have hoped. The fierce inner battle that happens from the time a person realises their true sexual feelings to the point where they come out is never ending. The battle is over and won after a successful coming out. For many this stage is not reached, they find themselves in a long term heterosexual relationship, or before they know it they are walking down that aisle and standing at the foot of the altar, married to someone of the opposite sex. Does this sound familiar?

This chain of events has usually been stereotyped in relation to men, who have struggled with their feelings towards other men and for one reason or another have found themselves married with children. There are many reasons; many have found this option far less daunting than taking the plunge and deciding to live life as a gay man from the outset. This is not exclusive to men however; it is something that happens to women too.

So what happens? We have discussed the feelings of knowing that you are different and then discover those feelings are an attraction to the same sex. During the teenage years he or she might have a limited sexual experience with someone of the same sex. In a fight to suppress these feelings and listening to external influences from respected family members, friends and peers they have been conditioned to think that these gay tendencies are a part of growing up, that it is merely a passing phase. Some even go as far as saying they are feelings of sexual discovery, a phase, a natural curiosity that will result in that person being fully heterosexual in time.

A common theme runs through those who come out as gay after they have married (as a heterosexual) - they've learned to suppress their true feelings, whilst having heterosexual relationships. There may have been the usual sexual activity like any other relationship or little intimacy at all. As they reach their twenties they decide to settle down, convincing themselves that they are straight, they might meet someone who they consider marriage material. This future spouse may have very little experience in the physical side of things and they are both unthreatened by one another. They marry, live as husband and wife and may go on to have children. For some this is a means to an end, they desperately want to have children, and feel this is the only way.

Somewhere along the line there comes the urge to change. This could be the manopause or menopause, call it what you will, nevertheless this is when the light bulb moment happens, then the realisation that the life they have chosen has been somewhat different to the one they wanted. A life changing event could also cause this reaction, a death, marriage difficulties, redundancy or a health scare. These are events that come with a lot of negative energy and stress and the only feel good factor comes from thinking "what if I did things differently".

As the children go through school and leave for University or to embrace their career the nest can seem bare and empty without them, this can bring on the realisation that it's you and the other half from now on. The gay husband or gay wife has now woken up to the fact that the marriage is no longer fulfilling them and begins to rediscover suppressed urges towards members of the same sex. This may lead to exploring the world outside the marriage perhaps frequenting gay bars, using the internet as an outlet to meet other gay men or lesbian women or perhaps beginning a relationship with a gay friend or colleague.

In time these new partners will be an addition to their existing life, these relationships no matter how casual will be enough to fulfil the need for the intimacy and understanding that they have spent so many years avoiding. However this only fulfils them for a period of time.

128

It is important to remember the health risks, not only should protection be worn at all times but there is also the mental health that can suffer. Is it fair to subject only a part of yourself to a life you want? Is it fair on your husband or wife to be cheated on because you could not express your true feelings before the marriage took place? It is understandable that you are hurting inside as you are unable to be the person you want to be, but think about the other person in this marriage. Do what is right for them too. If you are not happy this will inevitably make them unhappy in the long run.

What happens when you find that one person you fall in love with and you want to begin a relationship? I know this chapter is raising a lot of questions, probably only a few of the many questions you have asked yourself before.

Now comes the time to stop. You need to take a good hard look at the situation. This is not always easy to do alone, so speak to someone who can understand, perhaps a friend or a professional. They cannot give you the answer but use them as a sounding board and you will find the answer.

You may reach the decision that you wish to make the brave step and come out about your true feelings. You have been a long time in the closet and you are now sure that you want to take hold of the handle, open the door slowly and step out.

JEREMY ZHENG'S STORY

"I have been gay as far back as I have had memory, even as a young boy I knew I was attracted to my male friends. I never enjoyed playing with boys toys either, I was always happiest playing with dolls and girls but I was too young to indentify this as being gay. During my teenage years my family migrated to Australia from Vietnam, it was this change in my life that helped me to realise that I was gay. Living in Australia we are blessed with great weather and great beaches, it was on one of my first visits to the beach I spotted this red headed guy who took my breath away, all the signs told me I was gay. I would visit the news stands after

school and look at the gorgeous guys in Playgirl and flick straight to the male centrefold in Cleo.

I then became old enough to marry, it was expected. My mother's best friend showed me a photograph of her niece who was living in Vietnam. I told them I wanted to marry her; it was going to be a marriage of convenience. Convenient for me that is because she didn't speak English and then I could pursue relationships with other men. I went to Vietnam and married her and brought her back. I know this sounds so cold and selfish but I couldn't risk anyone finding out. On our wedding day I was desperately unhappy inside because I knew that it was going to feel more like a prison sentence than a life of wedded bliss. When she came with me to Australia she showed me so much love and respect I couldn't go off with other men, remaining married these eleven years never having ever been with another man. I have been a great husband and a fantastic father to our four children. We have three girls and a boy.

I knew then I would be living a lie and I know that I am living one now. I live in constant depression and decided I was going to end it all two years with an overdose. As you can see, it failed. My children witnessed me being rushed away in an ambulance to the local hospital. I didn't want them to have to go through that again and it is them that keep me alive. Out of all of this and with all my regrets, they are not one of them.

I now realise that I should have come out when I was younger. Coming from a large family, I am one of nine children; I lived with the constant fear of being disowned and rejected by my own family and this lead to the huge mistake of marrying a woman I didn't love to cover up my sexuality.

I would love to come out some day, to let those I love see the real me and to be accepted by everyone. The fear has switched from being afraid of what my siblings and family think to being afraid of what my children will think. It would kill me if I lost their love and respect.

Many men, and I suppose women too, marry in the hope that it will act as a cure or medicine to eradicate these feeling but it doesn't, in fact it

130

makes them worse. Nothing will make it better because you are not married to the person you truly love. I have never cheated on my wife, I have never had an encounter with another man, but I do know that I will one day. I have been speaking to a guy online from the UK who is visiting Australia next year and we plan to meet up. He is looking to migrate here and if he does then perhaps we could begin a discreet relationship.

My advice to all the gay men and women who are thinking of using marriage as a way to undo their sexuality is not to do it. It will never work, I am not being negative, it's just the truth. The pain and suffering of living in a marriage which is a lie is far greater than coming out and allowing your family time to adjust and get used to it.

Sex with my wife has always been difficult, having to find constant excuses to avoid sex or having to go through the motion whilst fantasising that I am making love to a man.

To conclude my story, I would like to offer some advice to parents who might suspect their child of being gay. Please be more open minded about the fact it might be happening to them. Be loving, caring, compassionate and kind to them. They are not unwell or diseased but just a bit different to everyone else, but it is not a bad thing. It is the good person inside that is important, not whom they choose as a life partner. Then mistakes like my own can be avoided, there will be no need to marry for convenience or attempt suicide as a way out. Living this life only torments my soul – not enrich it. I know that if any of my children come to me with issues about their sexuality they will receive my every support".

Coming Out

Coming out is not the easiest thing in the world to do, it comes with anxiety and uncertainty but it's something that many gay people face before they can live each day in the way that is right for them. This step of coming out will pretty much include what has already been discussed in Chapter Four; the only difference is there might be a husband or wife to consider and perhaps children too.

At the time you decide to sit your husband or wife down and explain your true feelings you will be at ease with your own feelings and sexuality. It is crucial to remember that although you have come to grips with it, they have no idea and they have to go through many emotions in order to come to terms with it. If they already suspect you might be gay it will come as a blow to them, there is a difference between thinking and knowing.

There are many ways to come out, it can either be gradually dropped into conversation by perhaps mentioning a gay friend that you know at work or another person you might know – it is important that the person you mention is someone you have not been intimate with. Perhaps steer topics that arise about homosexuality around to you giving a positive opinion or you are in support of gay culture. After a time it will then be easier to explain you have gay tendencies.

Another option would be to go down the route of sitting your husband or wife down and telling them outright. Make sure it is not done by blurting it out, just to get it over and done with. This is not the best way to get it out in the open. It is important to sit them down, make sure the children are away at the grandparents for the weekend or out for the day. It is important that your spouse has time to adjust to it.

There will be questions to answer, there are countless questions all of which will be phrased differently and the best answer is the one that feels right at the time. You can't revise for this, just control the situation so you can both remain as calm as possible.

- How long have you felt like this?
- When did you know you were gay?
- Why didn't you tell me before?
- Why did you marry me?
- Do you love me?
- Did you think about other men/women when we made love?
- Have you been with other men/women since we met?
- Do you have a lover at the moment?
- Where do we go from here?

132

Where indeed do you both go from here? Will your future consist of becoming great friends or does the marriage continue? If the marriage continues then it has to be for the right reasons, do not stay together for the sake of the children because that will make you both unhappy. It might be that by coming out you wish to make a new life with a new partner.

This is a massive upheaval for you both, although you have now made the courageous decision to show your true colours. There is a lot of history between you; you will still love one another because it was this love that united you both in the first place. Does the friendship that you both built together inside the marriage have to breakdown? Can you still continue to love and support one another but in the new life you have chosen?

It is important to keep a friendship if there are children involved this will make a happier home life for them, there will be change in their lives too, this can be limited if both parents maintain a good understanding of one another. Perhaps the gay spouse will want to move out or feel forced to move out. There have been couples who have established rules and continued to live with one another. This is not always possible for everyone. If it feels okay to stay and an understanding can be reached then surely this is best for all. If the situation is telling you both that it is time to part company with one another then perhaps this instinct should be followed.

The real answer is that it will be different for each couple. If the marriage continues then professional assistance might be required and the same should be said if the marriage is to end and there are children involved.

CRAIG O'NEILL'S STORY

"I am twenty-two and I have always known I was gay, as far back as I can remember perhaps seven or eight. Although I am a very open person, an open book some might say, that was the one thing I couldn't share freely with my friends and family.

I got through school by putting on a brave face, I learned the art of acting straight, some of my close friends saw through it but it was never discussed. When I was in school I had a girlfriend and with her being older it was seen to be cool. Knowing I was different from the rest of the school meant I kept myself to myself, this spilt over into my home life. It was a case of getting up, going to school, going home and staying in my bedroom waiting to be called for the evening meal. Then back to my room. Each day was a struggle. I enjoyed my own company then and I still enjoy it now.

When I was fifteen I had my first proper straight relationship, it was with a girl. She was great because I did care for her, but when you are gay, you are gay. This point in my life was a bit of a "catch 22" situation. I had an unhappy childhood and to be honest I couldn't wait to leave home. This was partly to do with my sexuality. I allowed the relationship to get serious so I could move out and break away from my old life and start anew. I felt a strong urge to live the straight life as it was not fair on my family to have to deal with the pressure of my being gay, so instead of coming out, I locked the closet door.

Three years past, I was still struggling with my true identity. My girlfriend had found out that I was gay during our first three years together. I had been having conversations with other guys on the internet, and she had found them. I was ashamed, and I was angry with myself for not removing the 'evidence' of my actions. I tried my hardest to change my feelings. I couldn't. It was brushed over and we carried on. Then we had our baby boy, Preston. The day he was born was the best day of my life, a feeling like no other in the entire world.

When Preston was eight months old, my girlfriend and I were having an argument and she stormed out of the house shortly after. I called my mum and asked her to make my bed up for me – I was going home. Enough was enough. Mum was frantically asking what had happened but I kept the conversation short. I just wanted to pack my life up and leave. Then my two sisters arrived, Chelsea and my half sister, Danielle. I told Chelsea I was gay, she said it was okay, I smiled and then I cried. I started packing my desktop computer, my girlfriend came back, my bags were packed and I was nearly ready to leave. She wanted to see the viewing history on the computer but I just wanted to get out of there. There was nothing to see anyway because I had wiped everything. I kissed Preston goodnight, then I left.

Living with her was not easy, especially after she had seen the activity on my computer. I know many would say "well who can blame her" but she had a chance to get rid of me there and then. But she didn't. Instead she would just wind me up and taunt me about my sexuality; she also went as far as saying that she would 'destroy' my life if I left her. She would tell everyone my secret, she even threatened me with this the day I left but by that point I was determined.

Now our relationship is strained. Even after I left she wanted me to stay and work things out. I had made up my mind and I came out to everyone. We hardly speak, even about Preston. I am there for him though, I have regular access and I am a main fixture in his life. He is my life.

Coming out meant I was free to be me. I am not proud of any of the things that have happened, my son excluded of course. A lot of people's hearts got broken including my own. I thought my world was about to end but there was light at the end of the tunnel and an indescribable weight had been lifted from my shoulders.

Being an openly gay man has made me a better person; I was in denial for a long time. I did question everyday after "Why did I do this...?" when I came out. As day after day passed by, I began loathing myself more and more. I hated myself and the fact that I had come out, mainly because my new revelation wasn't exactly met with open arms. But now it is better and well worth the heartache.

Don't get me wrong, I am not going to paint a picture that is perfect for you. My family still don't fully accept my sexuality. I feel awkward in certain situations, like when I am walking around the supermarket with my mum and a guy decides to check me out. It's uncomfortable although I do like male attention. My sisters and I are close, they are fine with it. Chelsea has been wicked, such a support and always 100 per cent behind me.

I do feel that I have been extremely selfish about living the life I have chosen. Or perhaps I should say that I have been selfish for the way I have lived my life. I am not proud to say that I did have experiences with other guys when I was still with my girlfriend. I did play it safe, it wasn't some random off the street, it was someone I had known for years and it just happened. It wasn't prearranged. I didn't visit the gay scene for some random pick-up because in all honesty I did not know that it existed, and when I did towards the end of my relationship I thought that it was a crime to go there.

They say that a wise man learns from his own mistakes, and a genius, he learns from the mistakes of others. Well, I would say this to all those gay men and lesbian women out there who are trying to fix everything by getting into a straight relationship or marriage. Don't do it. Live your life in the way you know is right and be the genius.

When I moved back to the family home I suffered an emotional breakdown, I was physically sick most evenings. I made an appointment with my doctor and explained my situation. I cried the whole time, I couldn't help but think she was laughing at me, obviously she wasn't. I felt stupid and ashamed of the person I had become. The doctor prescribed anti-depressants and sleeping pills and that really helped. It managed to stabilise my thinking as well as my sleeping pattern.

I feel that after all of my coming out experiences I have a well balanced life. I now visit the gay scene, quite regularly actually. In fact, I can't get enough of it sometimes. I have met so many wonderful friends who love me for myself and I know we are friends for life, especially my best friend Toby.

I will offer some advice about the gay scene though. When I first hit the scene I was a player, falling from one un-meaningful encounter to another, I guess it's called 'bed hopping' and again I am not being blasé about it and I am certainly not proud of it. I've hurt people and people have hurt me. I am a very forgiving person and I forgive them, I just hope they can forgive me too. I have changed and grown up a hell of a lot.

I wasn't born having a choice to be gay or straight. If I did then I might have followed the sheep that would choose the straight option for an easy life, who knows. As there is no option, who can say? If I could take a magic pill now, that would make me straight, I wouldn't take it! I am who I am. I'm Craig, Craig O'Neill, gay and proud to be so. If the word gay originally meant happy, then I am happy.

I now live with my boyfriend James in Worcestershire in the UK. We met by chance on FaceBook, I asked him out for a drink and he agreed. We met, and it was love at first sight. I knew he was the one for me. From that moment on we couldn't be apart, we would text or call each other all the time. We were like love sick puppies. We have been together for just over a year and we are strong now. Oh, it's not all plain sailing, James and I have had our ups and downs and we even split for two weeks but soon got back together – we just couldn't be apart. We learned that each of us needed our own space and now we are on the right road.

I now see Preston twice in the week and he stays overnight every other weekend. Preston and I, along with James are our own little family. I said earlier that some of my actions have been selfish and I suppose this time, my being selfish has paid off. I am settled now; I have a lovely home, car, son and partner. Preston will grow up to be a stable, well rounded individual who's dad just happens to be gay – he will grow up knowing no different.

I can't change the past but I do know that it has made me who I am today".

What To Tell The Children?

This is a dilemma; no parent would enjoy telling their child.

They will be shocked and slightly confused when they are told that either Daddy is gay or Mammy is lesbian.

Fundamentally it is up to you whether you want to tell your child, it should be a joint decision that will need to be discussed by both parents as there will be questions.

When a child understands this from a young age the effects are not as disruptive as when the child is older and begins to understand the dynamics of the world. This is when confusion starts and therefore careful answering of questions is required.

There are some things that might occur that will be beyond your control. There may be consequences at school if other children know about it. Children can be cruel and bullying might arise because of your coming out, it is important to make sure you speak to your child about school and if there are any problems, they must be addressed.

When a child who is in the midst of their teenage years or approaching adulthood discovers that their mother or father is gay or bi-sexual this can have severe effects on them, predominantly as they are going through a series of changes and going through their period of self-discovery too. This will unearth many feelings, emotions and questions. They see the world very differently until they go off and have experiences of their own, they may be resentful towards you and become homophobic as a result of needing to blame something for this change within the family.

It is important to get the timing right, the younger a child understands then it can begin to become accustom early on or you may want your child to go through the teenage years before they know.

The choice is yours and it is imperative to work through it with your spouse, so your child has an understanding that there is still a family unit even though you might not stay together. It should be done with the support of both parents; it should not be left to just one parent to deal with.

D.I.V.O.R.C.E

Divorce is the stage that indicates that the marriage is over. This is an unpleasant situation irrespective of the reason for the breakdown of the marriage; a series of emotions will arise that are necessary in order to deal with the divorce. It will require change from both husband and wife, as they part their separate ways and live their new life as they will come to know it. It might be a little bit easier for the spouse who is gay if they have already found a new partner; they will have begun to setup their new life so it is not as if both husband and wife are on an even keel.

It may not be so easy for the spouse who is left at home after the breakdown of the marriage because their husband or wife is gay. They now have to rebuild their life, picking up the pieces and trying to live a normal life, especially if left holding the children.

A positive mental attitude is everything at this stage, the feelings of anger, bitterness and anything that a person feels during this time is natural and understandable. These situations create a stronger person as a result and a positive future will evolve – but only if it is wanted.

THINK OF THE CHILDREN

Young children have a hard time dealing with the changes of divorce, we are forever told that consistency is hugely important as they grow and develop. It can be as difficult for older children too, it depends mainly on their age and their ability to understand what is going on. There is a loss of routine and family pattern, there will also be added questions about the reasons the marriage broke down. Regardless of age and maturity this situation will be difficult for all concerned.

It is imperative to bear in mind that you both brought your child into the world; therefore despite your feelings toward one another, it is important that the children do not experience too much change, get a fear of being abandoned, lose the bond with the gay parent and not witness arguments.

There are situations where the gay parent might break all ties with their child, this is very rare. This will have serious damaging effect as the child grows; this situation is not their fault. As the gay parent, if you feel that it is difficult to explain the situation, remain a part of their life and explain when they can understand. If your spouse decides that because you have chosen this path then you can follow it without knowing your child, unfortunately you need to tackle the situation through the court of law. You have rights and so does your child.

ADAM MCILHATTEN'S STORY

"I realised that I was bisexual when I was ten or eleven years old. I was aware that I was attracted to both sexes and I was okay with that. I had my first encounter with a guy in his teens when I was thirteen and then I had my first experience with a man when I was seventeen and I have had around twelve encounters with men in total.

I met my lovely wife, Wendy at college and we have been married for eighteen years. I was ecstatic on our wedding day, it was the best day of both our lives and I meant my vows when I said them. We now have two wonderful children. My wife knows I have feelings for men in fact I told her before we got engaged. She was curious and was interested in what I told her, but she was never upset as she had always known how I feel about her.

I have had experiences with men but these took place before I got engaged to my wife and I have not had any experiences since then.

I married my wife because I am bisexual, she satisfies all my needs she is my best friend, my lover, a wonderful mother to our children and she is everything to me. I don't understand why gay men or women marry the opposite sex in order to straighten themselves out or to make others
140

happy. The only people they are hurting is themselves and their spouses. I married my wife because we met and fell in love and we are still very much in love however, being bisexual also means there is a part of me that needs the interaction with other men and although I have never acted on these feelings, this is a battle I fight.

I occasionally look at gay porn; but that's it, I do not go to the gay scene or pick men up. It has never happened and never will happen. I have chatted to guys online and had cybersex; I have also had phone sex with certain guys - but this is not something I would do with just anyone. My wife doesn't know this, yes it would be hurtful to her to hear it and I do not consider it cheating. We have a great relationship, when we are out and we spot a good looking guy we will both comment and then end up laughing about it.

If I could take a magic pill that would make me straight, then I would possibly take it. Not because I am ashamed of being bisexual but because life would be easier if I could live the wonderful life I have without being shadowed by other feelings. I am happy with the choice I have made and I know I would not have been happier settling down with a man as opposed to a woman, therefore I know the choice I have made is right and I am happy with that.

I am very happy most of the time, but sometimes I do desire sexual contact with a man. I haven't had sexual contact with a man for twenty years, and it really isn't much of an issue most of the time. Masturbation, phone sex, and fantasy work for me, well at least it has for the last twenty years. I do sometimes fantasise about other men when I am making love to my wife and likewise I sometimes fantasise about other women, I have no intention of turning fantasy into reality. It helps that I have a great wife who is very understanding".

Things To Remember

Everyone's happiness is important, although you are the one looking to change the dynamic within your family and your personal life, it doesn't mean you must be miserable. On the other hand it does mean that as you are the only one who knows what is actually going on, you need to be responsible for how this plays out. Remember the following and it may go better than you expected.

- Don't cheat behind your husband / wife's back. You may actually get more support from them having not acted on your urges. You know what you are without having to remind yourself by cheating.

- If a relationship materialises with a lover whilst still married and you are still in the closet then ensure that protection is used at all times. Do not put your spouse at risk of sexually transmitted diseases such as HIV, Hepatitis and Syphilis.

- When you decide to break the news make sure you know what you want to say, create a calm peaceful environment and make sure there are no distractions. A weekend might be a good time if it's not a busy one or involves work, send your child off to stay with grandparents for the weekend. You will need this time to talk through everything.

- When it comes to the child there are two options to consider, tell them or remain vague about the situation. There is no right or wrong, you will know what is right. If they know and they do not reject you because of the truth then you can truly be yourself without worrying about prolonging the agony of when to tell them.

- Remain an important part of your child's life. Regular contact and the same amount of interest will need to be maintained even though you are no longer at the family home. If it is decided that you are the full time guardian of your child then make sure that the child spends equal time with both parents. They are not weapons.

RICK DALES' STORY

"I always thought in my pre-teenage years and then as I became a teenager that I was just going through a stage when I fantasised about playing with boys. I was lucky enough to have a friend who did as well so we played during "sleepovers". I always thought about playing with guys more than girls as a teen. During university I had the chance to have a few encounters with a guy but usually with the help of alcohol. I dated women because that was the natural thing to do and did enjoy sex with them as well.

Today I am married to my wife Jane, and we will celebrate our sixteenth anniversary this summer. Our wedding day was one of the happiest days of my life, that and the birth of my children, of course. I truly did love my wife and was happy to be marrying her. I do have an inner struggle now however. I didn't back then and figured that I would just overcome the odd feeling I had to be with a guy. Over the past few years, as my wife and I settled into our family life, I have struggled more with the feelings that I was in the wrong place in my life.

I have two wonderful daughters that I would give anything for. I have really struggled living my life the last couple of years. I still love my wife dearly and my kids are my world. I have found however that I am avoiding sex with my wife whenever I can because it doesn't do as much for me as it once did. I however have no plans on changing my marital status. There is no way I could tell my wife or my kids that I am leaving and why I am leaving. I have just become accustom to living my life with constant guilt.

There are times when I think my life would be easier if I came out. But, when I think of all the family and friends that I would be hurting (because they wouldn't accept it) I can't do it. It felt good when I told one person my true story but that was also because I knew that after we met on vacation and became instant friends that I would never see him again, once the vacation was over. He lives in England and I'm in Canada.

I have had experiences with other guys. Starting early in my pre-teenage years, I would play with them, meaning giving and receiving blow jobs, this went all the way to university. I have also been with a couple of guys since I have been married and gone as far as having sex with them but I have never been on the receiving end. I still struggle with that and to this day am not ready for it.

My advice for gay men who are looking to marry a woman but deep down truly desire men is to weigh all their options. Being gay is far more accepted in today's society than even ten or twenty years ago when I was contemplating marriage. They should be prepared that the inner struggle doesn't go away. I personally am shocked at how much the struggle has consumed me personally.

I don't think my children have been affected by this at all because I make sure my life seems like every other "normal" father in a "normal" family. My wife, however, is affected because I am sure she often questions whether or not I still love her. As I said earlier, I do, but it certainly isn't as strong as it once was and our sex life has become more of a chore to me than enjoyment.

I also suffer an internal battle because of my faith, I am a Christian yet many Christian beliefs tell us it is wrong for one man to desire another and that God created us as man and woman - to be partners together. I personally believe that the Church is incorrect in their doctrines but will probably never see the day that they accept that. We do have a gay Church in Toronto, but I attend Church with my family and they would never go there and I can't really tell them that I want to leave our Church to become a member there.

I do suffer through periods of depression (have since teenage years) and more often than not, those periods lately have focused on my state in life and not being happy with it. I suppress my feelings as deep as possible so they don't surface; it is a constant battle with myself. I stay away from our local gay scene because of the fear of being seen. Living in the closet means you can't let others find out or else the closet door will be blown wide open. When I have had encounters with other men it is usually through cybersex online and I have met up with a couple of guys in real life. One "relationship" has been on and off for almost one-and-a-half years now.

I was asked that if I could take a magic pill that would make me straight, would I take it. Although the answer might seem very obvious, to me that is a tough question. I don't think there is anything wrong with being gay or bisexual, however, given my love for my family (both immediate and extended) I would be tempted to say yes just to keep them from harm if my truth ever came out".

CHAPTER ELEVEN

Being Tagged And Stuck With The Pigeons

Gucci, Fendi, Prada and Louis Vuitton. We can't have enough labels, can we? We love them. We are not content in buying everyday things that have a label attached to them, we also feel the need to label and brand people we see in our communities. We humans like to treat each other the same as pigeons; we are tagged and sorted into groups. If you ran a survey, asking the average person on the street to describe a gay man or women there would be a multitude of answers. Some might say that the gay men would be good looking, smartly dressed and smell great, while others might say effeminate, flamboyant and love to gossip. As for the women, they may say attractive, tall and well dressed, while others might say butch, dress similar to men with shaved heads and flat shoes.

How many would actually say that they act and look just like everyone else?

The examples above derive from stereotypes, these are answers that people in the street might give and a lot more too, because they might associate a gay person with a character from their favourite soap or comedy drama, someone they work with or someone within the family who is gay. The fact of the matter is all the descriptions will be correct because as individuals we come in all shapes and sizes. We all have our own style of dressing, and we act in a way that makes us feel comfortable, this is what makes us unique.

Let's look at the Top 10 pigeon holes in which gay people have been incorrectly shoved into. Let's dispel the fairytales and provide clear answers. Here are some of the pigeon hole stereotypes that have formed people's opinion of the gay community.

Pigeon Hole:

"Gay men are effeminate bitchy gossips and all lesbian women are butch".

Fly, Pigeon, Fly:

This is a perfect example of how the gay stereotype has influenced others to believe that this is how gay people behave. Gay people come in all different shapes, sizes, ethnic origins and backgrounds. Stereotypes are created by taking the most memorable things about a certain type of person and then throwing them all together to create the image. They are usually over exaggerated. This is not something that happens to just gay people. Stereotyping can influence people's thoughts on other minority groups and individuals too. When you see a blonde woman you might automatically think 'dumb blonde'. You might expect them to talk slowly and seductively and have no intelligence or common sense. Upon meeting the person you may find out she is a very successful businesswoman. Stereotypes have been created by people like Marilyn Monroe and Dolly Parton. For all their blonde hair, these two icons were blessed with masses of intelligence and have used the stereotype to their full advantage. Some gay people will embrace the stereotype and use it to their advantage or they will go far away from it, to show that they are the exception. You must appreciate that the way you present yourself to the world has a massive effect on how the world perceives you. You are responsible for creating your own image, it reflects who you really are, and it goes hand in hand with the physical image and the mental attitude. Be true to yourself; make sure your outside matches the inside, so that you have an award winning image.

Pigeon Hole:

"Gay people are so promiscuous".

Fly, Pigeon, Fly:

This notion has come from a mixture of stereotypes and what others have observed around them. When I came out one of the first questions I was asked was "Why are gay people so promiscuous?" I found it to be a difficult one to answer. After my very first visit to the gay scene I noticed that there was little commitment and a great deal of promiscuity. Gay men are often promiscuous because they are either unable or unwilling to commit to a long-term relationship. Around 60 per cent of gay men are involved in a long-term relationship and a slightly higher percentage of lesbian women are. It comes down to what has been mentioned before, if you don't want a string of casual relationships or encounters then don't. If it is something you need to do in order to find your identity or discover your own sexuality then take care with your health as well as your emotions. It has been said that gay men have a similar number of unprotected sexual partners annually as straight men and women. I would have to say that protection is crucial. Unprotected sex in any relationship or sexual encounter should be avoided unless you are willing to deal with the consequences that unprotected sex can bring.

Pigeon Hole:

"You can't know you are gay when you have never been with a man/woman"

Fly, Pigeon, Fly:

This is very awkward to answer and the simplest way to answer is to throw a question to them asking "How do you know you are straight when you have never been with a man/woman?" We know how we feel inside towards the people we are attracted to. Remember you do not have to explain yourself to anyone.

As a living being we have a curious nature for experimentation. It would not be difficult to imagine that a gay man for example, who would consider himself categorically, 100 per cent gay to have a sexual experience with a woman. There are many reasons why a gay man or woman might have such an experience. Here are a few suggestions:

- They were trying to fit in with their peers and didn't want to accept that they were attracted to those of the same sex.

- They have a natural curiosity to see if they could be heterosexual and thought about people of the same sex while doing it.

- They called themselves gay and then realised that they are bi-sexual.

- They have had sex with someone of the opposite sex but did not enjoy it and do not feel any romantic interest for them but still see the beauty in them.

Pigeon Hole:

"All homosexuals will try it on with everyone they meet, even if they are straight".

Fly, Pigeon, Fly:

The automatic response to this statement from most people would be "Get over yourself". Although it is thought that this is a typical male response, I personally have heard just as many straight women say this as I have straight men. It has been said that homosexuality can make people uncomfortable or uneasy. It is different from what they class as 'normal' therefore they do not understand, and feel perturbed by it. They may feel that there is a chance that a gay man or woman might be attracted to them because they are of the same sex. It could be that they may not know many gay people therefore they have a stereotype lodged in their minds that gay people are sexually attracted to everyone of the same sex. The simple question to ask is, "Are all straight men/woman attracted to every woman/man they see?"

Pigeon Hole:

"In your relationship, who is the man and who is the woman?"

Fly, Pigeon, Fly:

This is interesting because society assumes that relationships have to include the more dominant, masculine partner and the feminine domesticated partner. This is a question I am frequently asked. Back in the day every man's home was his castle and the 1950's housewife had a meal on the table when he got home. Today, there are more career women who hold down jobs of equal or greater status to men thanks to Ms. Pankhurst and the Spice Girls – Girl Power! They don't have total equality irrespective of how much times have shifted. There are some house husbands now whilst the wife is the main bread winner. The relationship is a partnership and will only be successful if there is give and take on both sides. The crucial part is finding the right balance; we live in a world of infinite possibilities and equal opportunities. Does it matter who does the cleaning or who does the cooking? Does the person who vacuums the carpet take on the feminine role because the other washes the car? It doesn't matter.

Pigeon Hole:

"Gay people can't have a normal relationship like straight couples".

Fly, Pigeon, Fly:

If by 'normal' you mean getting drunk on Fridays and Saturdays, screaming and shouting and start throwing punches, then yes. If by normal you mean that you can be in a loving relationship, work hard, play hard and spend quality time doing the things you both enjoy, then yes. The workings of a gay relationship are identical to those in straight relationships; there are some people that view gay unions as inferior to heterosexual unions. Gay people fall in love and have long meaningful relationships. It is the responsibility of both individuals to ensure the relationship remains strong and succeeds, irrespective of gender.

Gay relationships can experience breakdowns, domestic violence and sexual problems and they get resolved in the same way as heterosexual relationships.

Pigeon Hole:

"All gay men want to be women and they all do drag".

Fly, Pigeon, Fly:

It is not a prerequisite that all gay men have to do drag. I have never adorned the frock and stilettos myself. It's something that hasn't interested me. If you want to throw on a glitzy little number and squeeze your size elevens into a pair of six-inch heels then do it. You don't have to do it, there are a few of my friends who have done it for special occasions such as Halloween and Christmas, and there are many other friends who share my view and have no intention of doing so. It is an artistic expression; it is celebrating the female form and adding the gay interpretation to it. We all know that women aren't really like drag queens; it's a flamboyant, over the top performance merely to entertain.

Pigeon Hole:

"Gay men are more likely to be child abusers".

Fly, Pigeon, Fly:

The comical thing is I have been asked about this directly, although it was not so funny at the time. It came from a colleague I worked with; it would be unfair on you for me to type what my response was to this small minded idiot but let's conclude that I made my point very clear. We are living in the 21st Century. I am fully aware that homosexuality is still not completely understood or accepted but it is an insult to assume that homosexuality is as perverse as child abuse. Being gay has no relation to paedophilia. Child abusers and paedophiles again come in all shapes and sizes; they are the people you queue with at the supermarket, or those passersby on the street. A female child abuser who preys on little girls is not a lesbian, they are a child abuser, and the same would apply if we were talking about a male child abuser who preys on little boys.

Pigeon Hole:

"AIDS/HIV are gay diseases".

Fly, Pigeon, Fly:

HIV can be contracted by any human being whether they are gay, straight or bi-sexual. Gay and straight couples who take part in unprotected anal sex have a higher risk of infection as the virus is transmitted easier and quicker because of the thin lining of the anal walls.

AIDS is caused by a virus called HIV which is the Human Immunodeficiency Virus. When a person is infected with HIV, the body will try to fight the infection and this is called being HIV-Positive.

Being HIV-Positive is not the same as having AIDS because the HIV disease wears down the immune system then the HIV will develop into AIDS.

It is crucial to have this understanding of HIV/AIDS in order to protect yourself from it. You can contract the infection from others who are also infected; you can, of course, contract the virus even if the other person doesn't know that they have it. It lives in the body therefore it can be transferred through semen, vaginal fluid, blood, and breast milk. It can be spread by:

- Having sex with someone who is infected
- Sharing a needle during the taking of drugs with someone who is infected
- Being born when their mother is infected
- Drinking the breast milk of an infected mother

The simple answer is ALWAYS wear a condom. This is a good protection against catching the virus during sex and don't share needles – kicking the habit is probably the best advice and make sure that needles are clean and disposed of properly.

For more information to those in the UK you can call the Sexual Health Line free (from the UK) on 0800 567 123 for help and advise or visit their website **www.CondomEssentialWear.co.uk**.

Pigeon Hole:

"Gay men hate women and lesbians hate men".

Fly, Pigeon, Fly:

It has been said that gay women are all man haters. Do you think this is true? I think not. The same thing has also been said about gay men, that they hate women. To begin with it is wrong to hate, it is a strong emotion and requires far too much energy. We would much rather put this energy into shopping. The gay women I know, to my knowledge, do not dislike men. I've yet to see them marching with placards chanting for their downfall and thinking about it, I can say the same from gay men on the subject of women. Most gay men idolise women especially those who fall under the title of Divas such as Bette Midler, Cher, Whitney Houston, Barbra Streisand, Liza Minnelli, Joan Rivers, Beyoncé, Kylie, Madonna, Cheryl Cole – I think I have made my point.

When I wrote this chapter I chose the Top 10 stereotypes and pigeon holes that gay people face. Then my cousin Debbie went and threw a spanner in the works, which was so brilliant I had to add it, although it was more a question as opposed to a statement.

This is my Plus 1

Pigeon Hole:

"There's no such thing as being bi-sexual!"

Fly, Pigeon, Fly:

My straight female cousin asked this because she has two best friends who are a male gay couple. She said one had never had any experiences with a woman and considered himself to be 100 per cent gay where his partner has had sexual relationships with several women in the past. It was an interesting conversation because it struck me that for a large part of my life I didn't believe in bi-sexuality. I thought it was black and white. You either fancy women or men. Obviously this isn't always the case; people fall in love or find certain people attractive. Others may explain it as liking classical music and heavy metal – they are totally different but one individual may appreciate both. Sometimes it is something that cannot be explained. So why try and explain it. It is what it is.

Bullying! Huh - Yeah! What Is It Good For? Absolutely Nothing!

Although we are at Chapter Twelve, this part of the book is just as important as Chapter One for me. I have written this book in some sort of sequence so it flows well and doesn't overwhelm you. I do believe that we have come to the point now where we need to discuss this. You may be dipping in and out of the book and not reading it in any form of sequence, again this is fine and your choice. The chapter you are reading now, for me, is the whole point of the book.

You Can Please Some Of The People Some Of The Time, You Can't Please All Of The People All Of The Time

You might look at your life and realise that you have spent a huge amount of your life worrying and caring about what others thought of you, think about the time and the emotional and physical resources you have wasted doing it. I know I have and could kick myself for it. Not that I am promoting self punishment, the time you have spent worrying whether people like you or not is dead time. It serves no purpose whatsoever.

You want to be liked and you also want to be accepted. Growing up we never want to be the last person to be chosen to play for a team. I say chosen, you are not chosen at all when you are the last one, you are merely the one that no-one wanted. School is a good primer for us to realise how many idiots there are in the world. In school we want to be accepted into a group or many groups, we want to make sure we fit in with the rest of the sheep, from our hairstyle to branded footwear; we want to look like everyone else. Many people break away from this when going to university, which is a great time to start experimenting with clothes, music, books, social circles and groups. Some people don't break away, they stay in the mindset that promotes the message that it is important to conform in order to fit in with the peer group, and those who have gone onto experiment will be noticed for their differences within society.

From the age of three I was incarcerated in an institution called School. I remained there until I was eighteen years old. It's lamented by many that 'Schooldays are the best days of your life' for me they were the worst. It's all about experience, I guess. I must admit that sending your child to school is probably the cruellest thing you can do. As it is the law of the land and I had wonderful, caring parents who had an appreciation that I must gain an education, therefore I went. I very seldom use the word hate, but I hated school.

The greatest lesson I learned is that kids can be cruel, and what I learned as I worked through my education is that cruel kids grow up to be cruel adults. There are exceptions, some of them have managed to get their act together and some have not. Bullies are highly skilled in turning a positive mood into a negative one in an instant, they leave us feeling lonely, vulnerable and with little self-worth.

How do I know this? I am not ashamed to admit I was bullied for pretty much all of my time at Primary and Secondary School. The earliest memories I have are being ignored, called names and just used as an object of scorn because the rest of the class felt like it. I always knew I was gay and never told a living soul until I met Andrew. People obviously knew, I didn't shout it from the roof tops; I couldn't say it to myself let alone tell others. It was as if they all knew, as if they could read my mind.

In Primary School I was in a class of around twenty-two kids, six of us were boys and the rest were girls, I learned that girls were bitchy and the boys could be twice as bad. They taunted me, called me horrible names, ignored me and were just cruel. Many years have passed, but I can still see their faces, hear their voices and recount their hurtful words. One vivid memory I have, I can still picture myself, what I was wearing, where I was sitting and who was there. If you don't think I know how you feel then believe me I do. I do appreciate that the things you were called and the times you were ignored are permanent scars that never heal.

When you have been bullied it can affect you at any point of your life, it can hinder you from mixing with your friends, creating a loving relationship, strip away the confidence to get the job of your dreams.

Why Do People Feel The Need To Bully?

Bullies are only comfortable and secure when everyone around them is miserable and insecure. They are at their height of happiness when they have chosen a victim, this person is more often someone who doesn't fight back because they are not emotionally or physically strong enough and might be different because of religion, race, sexuality or a disability. It might be hard to understand why a bully might not have compassion for others, as a child I was always taught that if you saw someone who was less fortunate than yourself then you help them if you can and remember "there for the grace of God go I", this is something that eludes a bully, there is no compassion or consideration. I am of the opinion that there are three types of bullies.

THE BULLY IS A VICTIM TOO

The abuse, torment and undermining stems from the bullies insecurities and unhappiness. A notion you might hear time and time again is the bully might in fact be a victim of bullying themselves. It maybe at home from a parent or sibling, it could be from another class member at school, or if you are an adult, from a colleague at work or from a bully who might be part of a social group or club. The bully might not have the strength to talk about their experience; therefore they work through their torment and regain their confidence by finding a new victim. There is a lot to be said about that, and it makes perfect sense, although it is of little comfort when aimed at you.

The bully's hostile home life might cause them to gain the power they lack at home by making someone else feel insecure and worthless. Perhaps the bully has forceful and insensitive parents; very little positive discipline, little or no affection and perhaps even violence.

159

These are things that you thankfully might not have encountered. If you were to imagine for a moment that you had this environment instead of the loving and caring home life you were fortunate to be blessed with, then you can at least understand why a bully can only communicate through negative talk and violent actions. As well as being victims ourselves because of their misery, they are also victims where there is a lot of upset and resentment towards anyone who has what they lack.

BULLIES ARE LIKE WILD ANIMALS

There are bullies that have no threat of becoming the victim they have a deep rooted personal pride, and need to show off in order to impress friends or establish status. It's a bit like in the animal kingdom where some species will fight all the males, to gain status giving them the right to mate with all the females. Translating this to the bully, may make you wonder why you were such a threat to them. Not only are they barking up the wrong tree but they are in the wrong forest!

THE BULLY NEEDS A FOOTBALL (OR A BARBIE DOLL TO PULL IT'S HEAD OFF)

This is short and sweet, it might be that these people just get their kicks out of using others as a football, and I don't mean that in a physical sense, they enjoy nothing more than causing torment and misery and there is no reason why they do it. You might be just another toy; something to get their kicks out of (pun intended). Just remember, people get bored of toys that aren't fun anymore, so don't react to their bullying and they will get bored of you, and move on.

When You Are Being Bullied

It is never easy when you have to admit that you are being bullied. Bullying can be administered in many different ways and there doesn't need to be any physical contact at all. It is surprising how many people believe that the definition of bullying is to cause someone physical harm. There are many forms of bulling in addition to name calling and physical assault.

These are:

- Being criticised in front of your peers
- Being deliberately excluded from a group or ignored
- Being and feeling undermined
- Being the subject of rumours
- Being taunted into doing something that you are not comfortable doing
- Being the subject of fun in a group where the only person not having fun is you
- Being made to feel undervalued and worthless
- Being blatantly whispered about while you are stood there or within ear shot
- Having your personal possessions stolen or hidden from you
- Being physically attacked with a fist, a foot or an object

When You Are Not Being Bullied

Although the above list is comprehensive it is our responsibility to recognise when we are the victim and when we are not. You need to establish the difference between friendly camaraderie and bullying. Whether you are gay or not it is natural for friends to banter and throw insults with no malice intended. I am sure the way you behave with your friends would not be acceptable in the way you would greet an acquaintance in the street. This is where rapport comes in, you will know the difference between a friend having a joke, and a stranger or acquaintance purposely going out of their way to victimise you. The reason I mention this is that there might be a misunderstanding, sometimes we hear what we want to hear and mistake what was said, depending on our mood. If you are spoken to in a way that does not sit right with you then you need to address it to give the other person an opportunity to explain what they have said, which may clear up any misunderstanding.

What Can I Do About It And Where Does The Buck Stop?

The types of bullying that have been listed are all the things I was subjected to at school. Yes, even being physically attacked with an object, in my case it was an art knife. I am not going into all of that now; I have saved that for Chapter Seventeen. It all happened a long time ago and it has been laid to rest now.

Today's bullies show much more imagination and enterprise, we now live in an age where if you can't shout or even whisper abuse to the victim then it can be done through emails, text messages and through social networking websites.

If you feel that you are the victim of bullying then I urge you to consider the following steps in guarding your safety. This is something I wish I had done and didn't because I had no one to suggest it and in hindsight carrying out these few simple steps could have actually helped:-

- Keep a record of all incidents such as date, time, location and how it was done and who was involved – were there any witnesses?

- Keep any emails, text messages and messages on your social networking page. It is far easier to press the delete button, I know, but running away from it will not help.

- Get strength and support from your friends if you can open up to them. They can be a great help and re-build your self-esteem when the bully decides to take a bit of it for themselves.

- You could approach the person who has treated you unfairly. I know just reading this your stomach has probably dropped. In most cases people don't know they are bullying, they might be taking their frustration and anger out on you and not even realising it. If you are confident and comfortable to approach them, then do it. Don't go in all guns blazing, just calmly approach them and explain how they are making you feel. They may not realise the distress they have caused, once you have addressed the situation you can both move forward. You may not be best friends with them however as they realise the effect of their actions they might put their energy into something more positive. If you have taken the brave step to address the bully and they are aware how they are making you feel then your happiness depends on you asking for help outside of the situation.

- You may genuinely feel that you cannot approach them, ignoring the situation will not help it go away; the answer could be involving someone outside of the situation. If you are being bullied in school then speak to a parent. I did this, it does help. When parents make contact with other parents then this can be an effective way to resolve the situation.

- You might want to discuss the situation with your teacher. We all have a favourite teacher at school, I was fortunate to have a few and could speak openly with them and have a laugh at the same time.

After Speaking Out

When you have spoken out the bully is defenceless as their power relies on them being undetected, once the bully's cover is blown, you have gained control of the situation. The bully is dealing with a situation that they had not factored in - having to explain their despicable behaviour.

I remember on one occasion I was being unusually disruptive in class and of course I was asked to stay after class. I wasn't a bad pupil and that is why I was asked to stay back, when we got down to it I mentioned that I was having problems with certain people. The teacher spoke to them and explained the situation and that if it continued then punishments would be handed out. From memory it was a group of people that were less threatening to me, they apologised and even though we didn't become great friends, it was a lot more pleasant when I saw them.

Remember the teacher is not just there to teach and mark your homework, they have a duty of care for your safety and well-being as well as making sure that there is harmony. I have massive respect for teachers and the work they do, especially in today's society, having to deal with hundreds of children and teenagers who are strong willed and have little respect for figures of authority. It is the teacher's role to speak to the bullies and their parents if necessary and issue immediate punishments or monitor the situation should a punishment not be immediately issued. It does work, so chose the teacher who you can talk to and have confidence in.

Bullied For Being Gay

It is a complex situation to admit you are being bullied simply because you are gay and you haven't come out yet. You feel that you have two options, either carry on suffering in silence or feel as if you are forced to come out just so you can deal with it head on. For you it is a lose / lose situation in that neither option is pleasant. I urge you to speak to someone. I was in the same situation; the only thing I could do was explain to my parents that I was being bullied. I explained to my mother that I was being called gay and that everyone was of this opinion, I told her that I wasn't. At the end of it all I was sixteen years old when the bullying stopped, I hadn't had a relationship with a female or a male although I knew I was gay. I had no attraction towards women. As I had not experienced a relationship with a man then I saw no reason to come out until it happened and I was hoping it would never happen. I wasn't looking for love and I was quite happy if it wasn't looking for me. All I truly wanted was to grow up being as happy in school as I was at home. Unfortunately a privilege I didn't have. For me the only relevant fact was I was being bullied, it didn't matter what the reason was, and the important thing was I was a victim of bullying and something needed to change. I didn't have to tell my parents what they were saying, I could have been vague with the truth, but I had to tell them so they could understand my situation. You do not need to tell people what they are saying, they are just using vile words to bring you down and they have no right to do this.

It is quite normal for those who are suffering homophobic bullying not to talk to anyone about the abuse they are suffering at school, in fear of being 'outted'. Homophobic slurs are also used to bully those who are heterosexual also, it is quite common now for things that are considered to be different, unpopular or 'uncool' to be referred to as 'gay' so by telling your parents or teachers about the language they are using you are not confirming anything about your sexual orientation.

If you are happy to open up to your teachers or parents, that you are being victimised because you are gay then I would suggest that you take the matter all the way if you do not get the outcome you want. Your school have a legal obligation to look after your safety. I don't recommend that you come out about your sexual orientation in school, you might want to at home but at school it is much different. Bullying usually stays within the confines of the year you are in, but when you come out the news will travel fast and your sexuality will be opened up to the entire school. I know this because a pupil in the year below me came out and the only thing I could do was stand by and feel sorry for him, he threw himself well and truly into the pit of wolves.

SEAN WADDEN'S STORY

"I knew I was gay when I was going into seventh grade; it marked the change between Elementary School, and Junior High. I remember thinking how exciting it would be to be able to finally take showers in gym class - and then I wondered, why would I want that to happen? Although it took me years to accept that I was gay, that was the one defining moment when I knew I was, even if I could hide it well.

I have not been bullied much for being gay, especially now I am in college. I am a pretty masculine gay, not many people suspect I am gay until I tell them. I have only had a single incident really. In High School there was a group of trashy kids that everyone called the Dirt Bike Kids. They were your typical bigoted rednecks, but pretty much left me alone - I was popular so they just ignored me. One day one of these kids called me a fag, so I blew him a kiss in response. He didn't take kindly to my response and wanted to try and fight me. I was not about to get suspended, so I just told him to calm down, not to get his panties in a bunch, however the situation escalated when ten of his redneck friends joined in. I started to walk away, when one of them grabbed the front of my shirt and went to punch me. My friend Nate then jumped him - started to fight, but a teacher broke it up. I was sent to the Principal's office, and I was going to be the one getting in trouble because I blew the kid a kiss, and I should know better. The next day I walked into school, everyone of course had heard what happened, but many people were wearing home-made shirts saying phrases in support of gays. Almost all of the students had made shirts, and were pissed off I was going to get in trouble. That day the Principal talked to me, saying he had thought it over and I was not going to suffer any consequences.

I told my parents I was gay, and I was not allowed to attend school, nor allowed out of the house. I had to go see a therapist to work on not being gay. After two weeks of this, I told them I was confused, and that I was cured. I'm sure they are more accepting now, but I'm not telling them until I graduate college. I feel like they do not deserve to know that part of me, to really know their son because they rejected me. I get along great with them, as long as being gay is not mentioned. I still live at home, and go to school full time, so I really have to rely on them.

The gay scene is something I sometimes dislike. Saying this there are times I love it. The substance abuse and unsafe sex that goes on I find wrong and it gives the gay culture a bad name for being promiscuous and disrespectful to ourselves and others. I am anti-drugs and I am disgusted they have become such a problem within the gay scene, they are everywhere. Unsafe sex is extremely dangerous in this day and age, especially within the gay community; if more people were sensible then AIDS would not be as prevalent. Getting some of the dislikes out of the way, I find that gay people are almost always the nicest, most caring people and I rarely find a gay person who is horrid and bigoted. This is something I am extremely proud of; there are no other groups out there who can boast that".

Bullying In The Workplace

Bullying does not stop in the school yard; it can either carry on or even start whilst at work. You may have gone all through school and not
166

have encountered a bully until you have reached the workplace. Remember, bullies come in all shapes, sizes and ages therefore the same principles apply.

The same as the teacher, it is your employer's responsibility that you work in a happy, safe and friendly environment so that you are not discriminated against in any manner.

In actual fact there are more laws to protect you from being bullied as an adult than when you were a child. Any form of discrimination can be reported to your union or the company's Human Resources Department who will offer free and impartial advice. It is probably not a good idea to rush off to your union or HR department to resolve the matter, again there is a need to deal with this situation calmly and sensitively – with your line manager or professional body.

- In the first instance if you feel that you can deal with the situation yourself then ask for a moment of the bully's time and explain to them what they are doing and how this makes you feel. Keep to the point and explain yourself clearly. You might want to do it on a break time or on a lunch hour. The timing is crucial, do not plan to do it as you are about to be whisked off to a meeting, it is important that it is not rushed. There are sure to be questions that you will both want to ask.

- If you feel that the matter has not been resolved having spoken to them or if it gets worse, approach the manager that you have performance based meetings with or another senior person who you feel might understand, they can then bring you and the bully together to act as a mediator.

- Should this matter persist then it is now time to take the matter to your union representative or Human Resources advisor.

Since coming out I have come to the point that I can have a laugh and a joke about who I am, and I am proud to say that people find it very easy to laugh and joke with me without having to worry about offending me. I find those people who are politically correct to the point of

167

ridiculousness extremely amusing to talk to. You can just see them tip toeing and skirting around what they are saying in order not to offend and then if you say something off the wall about gay people then they begin to look at you as if you have bashed them over the head.

I did have an experience in a previous company where a member of the management team, whom I knew more as an acquaintance rather than a friend said something to me, and for the life of me I cannot remember what it was, I only remember it really infuriated me. I had many choices in the way I could deal with this. I could have approached him directly, I could have gone to his manager or I could have gone to Human Resources. I felt comfortable handling it myself - I chose an appropriate instant to ask for a moment of his time. I explained that whilst I didn't take myself or my sexuality too seriously and I am happy to have a laugh and a joke, his comment went too far. He explained that he didn't realise that he had crossed the mark and he apologised and we carried on. I found it hugely important not to play the sexual discrimination card; we were both adults and it just needed to be mentioned so we could reinforce the boundaries.

A well respected company, who cares about their employees as much as they do their bottom line, will want a happy work force who feels safe and comfortable in the working environment.

NEWSFLASH: There Is Life After Bullying

Bullying doesn't come with a shelf life; it can be something that lasts for days, weeks, month, years and even a lifetime. The duration is very much up to the individual's tolerance towards being bullied, it could end just as quickly as it started or if you have a high tolerance then you can live with it for years and years. Even when it has stopped, it stays with you for the rest of your days. It can sometimes happen just before you form a friendship. How many times have you been introduced to a group of people to find that there is one or two that just seem to be on another page to you? As you get to know them you realise that although they are different they are good people and you like them for their diversity. I know I have done it, you shouldn't judge a book by its cover.

168

Bullying is negative; the things that we are told and made to believe become ingrained in our sub-conscious mind which has a negative effect on our self-esteem. When we beat ourselves up by calling ourselves stupid and worthless, we are reassuring ourselves that we are all those things the bully once said to us. Using the exercise in Chapter One will help you easily eradicate these negative feelings and then break the pattern of self-talk. You know you are not stupid and worthless; these are the powerful effects that happen when you allow a bully to store negative rubbish in your sub-conscious.

There are people out there who have been so badly bullied and for so long as children, that they are still affected by it today, although they are now adults and the bullying has stopped. I know that these people may have low self-esteem, low self-worth, little or no confidence and suffer with nervous disorders or panic attacks during problematic situations. There are those who have been so affected that depression and anxiety can set in along with thoughts of suicide. I don't have to remind you that suicide is a permanent solution to a temporary problem.

Victims of bullying may:

- Have a paranoia that people are talking about them
- Avoid social events and gatherings and become reclusive
- Have trouble talking or holding conversations with others
- Have problems with trusting other people
- Avoid striking up a new relationship with a partner
- Avoid striking up a new friendship
- Have no career aspirations due to a lack of self-belief
- Have a need to be severely self critical of themselves and others and quick to blame themselves
- Find it difficult to control their emotions as they are overwhelmed by certain situations
- Be negative in general and always looking for the negative instead of the positive
- Avoid fun situation in the belief they will only lower the mood
- Avoid interaction with groups they want to be a part of

Change For The Good

I became a recluse during my teenage years; I didn't want to go out, see anyone or speak to anyone. The only social life I had was with my parents, we had such fun together but in terms of friends, I didn't have any. Was it the right thing to do? In hindsight no, I should have tried harder to find people I could relate to and I should have made myself go out, my experiences of people had left a negative effect and unconsciously thought that most people were rotten and now know that so many are not.

Do the things YOU want to do. You only have one life and you should enjoy it the way you want. This can be whatever works for you; for me it was listening to a certain genre of music and for a close friend of mine it was getting absorbed in movies that helped her through clinical depression, so there is a lot to be said about 'a little of what you fancy does you good'.

You may have been treated badly by those who have no rights to speak to you the way they did, the things they said might be cruel and hurt today as much as they did when they were first said to you. By giving up on the things that you want to do you are letting them win. This may stop you from going on to further your education, or a professional apprenticeship or pursuing a hobby. You might just be sat at your place of work, looking at the career ladder, too afraid or just unresponsive to take the step onto the next rung. It is only when you start living the life that you deserve, and truly want that you will be truly happy and fulfilled.

SANDRA BURTON'S STORY

"I was around the age of ten when I began noticing I was different to the other kids, but didn't really think much of it until I was twelve.

I was severely bullied growing up as very few people believed in gay rights. I got the name calling, whispers in the yard that I could hear as I passed by and just being made to feel like garbage. I was extremely lucky that the friends I had were quite powerful in my school, and they stood up for me. I could handle the bullying as I was not willing to take anyone's crap.

Coming out was hard to say the least, before I decided to tell a person I first asked "What do you think about gay people?" and if they were fine with it, I'd tell them. I actually had to get one of my friends to tell my homophobic friend for me because he used to talk about how homosexuals should be beaten to death. As it turned out, my homophobic friend changed his mind when he found out about me, and started accepting it.

I am not fully out of the closet yet, but I am half-way there. My close friends know, I have to be careful as it is a homophobic school. A girl that I knew (she's older, so this happened before I reached High School) came out and told people and she lost her whole circle of friends. I know I can't tell my family or they would kick me out. So I just go along telling person by person but only those whom I trust.

It is just as scary telling the next person as it was the first, I would have thought that it might get easier but it doesn't, you just don't know how people are going to react. I was afraid in the beginning that if people knew or found out then they might beat me to death.

Coming out to the trusted few has been the best thing I have done, however it is frustrating not being able to tell people who I really am, being gay seems to be a very controversial topic. I hear many people say "oh, that's so gay" or talk about how they hated gays, lesbians, bi-sexuals and transgender and to be honest it terrifies me. When I did tell people, some people stopped talking to my face and started talking behind my back. Some people told me that I was disgusting, and some people stayed true to me. Everyone has their own way of dealing with stuff like that, I suppose.

I am suffering an internal battle with my sexuality and my religion, I was born and raised as a Catholic and my faith doesn't look kindly on what I am. I feel that I am misunderstood by my family, some friends and also my faith.

My friend is bi-sexual and although we are not dating, we hold hands when we walk around town, we get a lot of people staring, whispering and giving us bad looks. We hold our heads high as we have nothing to be ashamed of. She's the main person who gives me confidence in my sexuality. When I'm with her, I don't care about what others think because she's what gives me hope the next morning. She's always there and knows what goes through my head. People can stare and talk as much as they want, because when it comes down to it, they're not the ones that are going to stand by my side - she is".

Picture Power

Having bad memories playing out in your mind is unpleasant, these can be the result of bullying or being caught up in a bad situation - a situation that given a choice you would never have experienced. These thoughts are always there, sure you can distract yourself, they go away, then they make yet another appearance and this process changes your entire mood. There is something that you can do about this. This is another one of the techniques I discovered when studying for my NLP (Neuro-Linguistic Programming) Practitioner qualification.

Try this to help those memories you could do without.

1. Close your eyes and think of a favourite memory, something that makes you feel good and safe, a strong memory. It can be anything, and it will either be running in your mind like a movie or just a still shot, like a photograph. Just breathe and look at the picture in your head and notice how you are feeling. You feel good.

2. Now turn up the volume so it's comfortable to listen to and set the colours in the picture to how you want to see them, make it as bright or as soft as you want. You can put it on replay so it never stops and you can adjust the speed that is right for you. Do it as you would when you adjust the volume and colour settings on your television. You are feeling great now.

172

3. Now think of the memory that upsets or hurts you. Again this memory can either be running in your mind like a movie or just still like a photograph. Just break and look at the picture in your head and notice how you are feeling. You are fine, it's only a memory and it holds no real harm to you.

4. Now, turn down the volume so you don't have to hear the sounds associated with this picture. And now turn down the colour so the colour drains from it, it will now look like a black and white photograph or it will be running like one of those black and white movies they show on a Sunday afternoon.

5. Now to complete this, you have to take the bad colourless memory and squash it until it's really small, pushing one side in at a time. Make it as small as you can. Now, we need to replace it, so take your good memory and throw it on top of that black and white object and now you are left with your first memory in tact. Breathe in and take a good look at it. Notice the colours, the noises associated with it; make the picture bigger if you want, more colourful, more noise. If you don't it is fine. But the good memory has now destroyed the old memory. It's gone. You are now left with the happy memory.

This will work for any memories you want to put to the back of your mind. Of course it will still be there, this technique cannot wipe your mind but it will not jump into your head so frequently, if at all. It's power has decreased, you have removed your association with it and it has no control over you or your emotions.

Do It Alone Or Have A Helping Hand?

There are choices available and there is life after bullying. There are those who will always remain the victim because it is easier to blame others for inflicting the pain, and then blame themselves for being the terrible person they were told they were. There are those who have made the conscious decision to pick themselves up, dust themselves off and then stick two fingers up at those who are insignificant in the cold light of day.

You don't have to do it alone. It may surprise you to learn that there are people out there who can assist you to become the person you want to be. It is perfectly achievable to be the person you want to be and get the life you want. Now, this will vary depending on individual needs, this can range from the Mental Health Team to Life Coaching.

When I was growing up I thought I needed counselling. I lost my Grandmother at a young age which had a profound effect on me and although I had two phenomenal parents whom I could talk to, I believed I needed a counsellor and I never spoke to my parents about wanting one because I though it would be a sign of weakness. I often wished I had someone independent of the family I could have spoken to.

During this process of self-discovery you will lay your troubles about the times you were bullied to rest, especially if they have been suppressed deep down inside hoping they will never resurface again. It can be a painful experience but it will allow you to remove the weight from your shoulders that you no longer need to carry. Keeping the bully alive inside will eat you up and restrict you in ways that you could not have thought imaginable. Let it go. Give yourself the opportunity to forgive the past and those who have wronged you and move forward to a life that others will envy. It is important that you speak to yourself with respect. If I was to meet you, and I called you the names that you call yourself, would that be right? If it is unacceptable for me to speak to you in that way, what makes it right for you do so? When you talk to yourself, be kind and think about what you are saying to yourself.

Whether you decide that you wish to take on the services of a Counsellor or a Life Coach is entirely your decision. Any respectable professional would offer a free consultation in order for you to see if they are right for you. This can be done face to face or via the phone. My clients have experienced fantastic results either way, and the feedback has been astounding. Most clients prefer the phone, as they can fit their coaching time in during a lunch break or before they start work or after they finish. There is no travelling and it can be done from your own special place at home, or outside, you are in complete control. To get a great Life Coach or Counsellor ask around but be sure to use a professional body member, someone who has been accredited.

174

The majority of my clients come through word of mouth, you are more likely to trust those who have used the service than believe an advert created by the professionals themselves. Read the testimonials that have been written by existing and past clients as they are a great indicator to the type of service you will receive.

Life Coaching along with other alternative therapies is a great bonus, using proven techniques such as NLP and Hypnotherapy can elicit long term relaxation and can help with refocusing on what is important and letting go of the things that are not. We all need a spring clean every now and again. Think of that time when you decided to ransack through your old clothes and those DVD and CD collections so you could list them on eBay. Well sometimes your subconscious needs clearing of the rubbish that is stored in there. Don't think that NLP and Hypnotherapy can only cure bad habits, phobias and fears. It will improve in the areas where you are lacking, you will feel re-energised and re-focused and you will see instant results. Once again true professionals will offer a free consultation in order to assess whether it is right for you and also right for them too. It is a two way relationship. If they cannot help then they should point you in the right direction.

Open Surgery

As you know I am NOT a doctor therefore I cannot give any medical advice. I mention this from my own personal experience. You are your own person and you know your own mind therefore this is just to enlighten you on someone else's situation. In this case it is my own.

Should you feel the need to visit your doctor, he or she may prescribe some type of medication such as anti-depressants for anxiety or depression. After the years of torment I received through school, then a change in my circumstances with my parents moving abroad I was diagnosed with depression. I didn't know I was depressed, the change hit me one morning, the only way I can describe it, is it was like a tidal wave, it just hit me. I felt sad, scared, vulnerable and so very, very alone. Over a period of two weeks I went to bed each night and dreamt that someone close to me had died. One night my mother, the next night my Dad, the night after my sister-in-law and so on, it went on and on. I went from a healthy 12.5 stone to 11 stone and I didn't know it at the time but everyone close to me was worried. It was only after I came out the other side my family told me how worried they were. I was eating, Andrew made sure of that, but whatever I was eating just got churned up inside me. I would go to work as normal, and found myself going to the toilet so I could cry. That was all, I just needed to cry. I then went to the doctor and he told me I was suffering depression and immediately wanted to prescribe anti-depressants. I told him politely that I would not take them, and I didn't need them. I explained that I didn't even take pain killers for a headache so there was no way I was going to take them. He said he would refer me to a Counsellor, I heard nothing for six months, during that time I battled every single day because I was determined to get my life on track. I did it. I had Andrew to help me and a few close family members and I made it through the other side. It was the hardest battle of my life. It went as fast as it came.

I understood that I would not have been weak in taking the anti-depressants; I just knew I had enough fight inside me to get over it. I kept a positive mental attitude each and everyday, it was an uphill struggle, taking one step at a time, I realised that if I kept climbing there was only one way to go. Anti-depressants are not a sign that you are defeated and neither is depression. It is a stage you go through in order to come out stronger. With anything you need to admit there is a problem there, once you come to terms with it, you can deal with it. It was my personal choice whether I took the medication, and I chose not to. I was more worried about the fact I was so upset each and everyday, and the fact I could not go to bed without the nightmare of losing someone else. Once the doctor had diagnosed my problem I was ready to fight because I knew what I was dealing with. I also knew that by refusing the medication that Andrew would give me the extra support to get me back on top. After I combated my depression I was then told by a colleague that he was on anti-depressants, I was shocked because I had no idea that he was struggling with depression, it helped him to become more balanced and to keep control. In any event, always discuss it with your doctor.

I hope my sharing this with you helps you to realise that there are others out there that have been bullied, that have felt the adverse and long term effects of it and with a willingness to let it go, you can be freer than you ever imagined possible.

Let it go.

There Is Always A Moral To The Story

Bullies look no different from the rest of us, they blend in well with conventional society; they aren't actually nasty to everyone. Bullies have feelings too, they love and care for people and people also love and care for them in return. The bully does what he or she does because they are either a victim themselves, or feel threatened by something they don't understand. It could be they do not understand the differences in a person's culture, faith, sexuality, origin, or if the person does not conform to the social 'norm'. It might be that the person is not the right size or shape, has a set amount of finances, wears the correct fashion, and has a different hair colour or not being born into the right social class. That is why so many people are bullied, we are each born different, we sometimes look the same but when you dig deeper we all have a different story to tell. If we just accepted people for what was on the inside instead of concerning ourselves with the tangible non-sense, then life would be far more enjoyable for all involved.

Another lesson I learned from school was that bullies are the minority. It's not easy to get your head around that one when you are being bullied; you are made to feel that everyone is against you whether you are in the school yard or at your desk in work. What you learn is that the bullies are the minority and the people who actually like you are in the majority. It is because you have withdrawn almost completely that you don't see it. You have removed yourself from the bigger picture therefore the only picture you are left with is the one with you and the bullies.

Open your eyes and look around, you will see that not everyone is against you. There are respectable, well mannered and well rounded

177

people in your school yard or in your office that you have never interacted with. You might have said hello to them while you were out and about and even held the door open for them; take time to get to know them and who knows what wonderful friendships might blossom.

EMMA CLARKE'S STORY

"I suppose I have always likes girls from a very young age, but probably didn't really understand this until I was around fifteen or sixteen. I waited until I was twenty-one until I decided to come out of the closet. That for me was the right time.

I had a tough time in school; I would get verbally abused with insults being hurled at me as I passed people in the corridors. I was also physical attacked, it's not something I really want to talk about, it is just too painful to have to go through. Being in the changing room for sports was the worst. I would get looks off the girl as if I had the plague. They thought I was going to try it on I suppose. I had no interest in any of the girls in my school. I then became friendly with a group that didn't even question my sexuality, it was unimportant to them. Sometimes if people were whispering about me or shouting abuse they would be supportive and we would just have fun. I realise now that those group of friends were not the most popular in school but they were the nicest. They looked a bit different with their black hair, dark clothes and their eye make-up; I suppose they would be called 'Goths'. Our group was a refuge for all those who had noticeable individuality.

I came out at the age of eighteen and having to come out what about as nerve wracking as it gets, I had been with a few women before coming out and a girl I spoke to on a website gave me the courage to come out, the two hardest people to tell were my best friend and my mother. My best friend was supportive and deep down I think she had a feeling I was. My mother didn't really believe me and thought I was going through a phase in my life; I assured her that it wasn't a passing phase. After those two it was very liberating to come out to everyone else.

It was actually better than I thought possible, most people were accepting and those who don't obviously don't care for me and as it is

178

such a big part of who I am, if they don't like it they can lump it. I am thankful that I have exactly the same relationship with my parents as before I told them, except now they may joke about hot looking girls. It is truly the best thing I have ever done.

I have left the past where it belongs, in the past. I can hear the distant echoes of their small minded jibes. My advice to anyone reading this right now who is getting bullied is get good friends, look and you shall find. Speak to your parents, you don't need to tell them what they are saying, don't suffer in silence and speak to your favourite teacher, we all have a favourite and they will be on your side.

I have a lot of wonderful friends, many of whom are straight. I love the gay scene too, and I have met some very nice people there, it is so different and extravagant compared to the normal straight scene. I feel at ease and comfortable when I am there and I like being a part of the gay culture. Just go with an open mind and keep your wits about you".

Social Networking Site Warning:

Many social networking websites come with a privacy and safety control so it is important to implement them where necessary so that you know who is viewing your personal information. You can also limit who can find you and communicate with you. Bullying only requires communication, so even though there is a computer between you, the effects can be just as horrible as if they were in the room with you. In fact, it can be worse as you are being bullied in the place where you should feel the safest, at home. If you are being harassed then you can block people from seeing your profile. You can report abuse and misuse directly to the website and they can deal with the matter and if you feel that social networking via the internet is not working for you then close your account, this can be done usually with a few clicks of a button.

Be kind to yourself and know when you need to be selective about the people you choose to socialise with.

CHAPTER THIRTEEN

Mental Health Check

Before I begin I will start by saying that I have adopted the Joan Rivers way of dealing with difficult situations, that is - laugh about them. It is far easier to talk about past events by adding humour. The other day for example, I was spending the weekend with a close friend who I have not known that long, you know, one of the people you meet and don't ever remember not knowing. We were both talking about depression; actually we started talking about body weight. I said that depression although it has a lot of bad press it is marvellous for weight loss (I was at my lowest weight during my depression, although at my weakest - I looked fabulous) and then I started to strut and pose. She burst out laughing and was in agreement as she suffered the ill effects of depression too and experienced the weight loss. She said that although she was severely depressed she looked amazing, again we both laughed – to the point where we couldn't breathe.

The next day I woke to the sound of the radio, there was a discussion on depression and a lady called to say her husband suffered depression and as a result he took his own life four days after Christmas in 2008. I was numb. The conversation from the previous day replayed in my head. I felt awful. This feeling stayed with me for most of that day, even though I was laughing about myself and not about anyone else - I felt dreadful.

Then I came to the conclusion that the way I handle personal situations is to laugh about them following the aftermath. It is the only way I can function without taking on the weight of the world. Perhaps in the same way that no matter how worthless I felt at the hands of the bullies at school, I remember that I always had a smile on my face. That smile was there for me, and it was there for the people that mattered to me. And it is where it remains to this day.

This chapter might be a little heavy however there is a lot of great advice to be had here so take it in your stride and keep smiling. You will progress through these pages effortlessly by taking it slowly.

Here We Go

It has been estimated that around one in every four people have suffered or will suffer with depression, the most frightening statistic is that in the UK around ten percent of children have a mental health problem at any one time. Depression is a mine-field as this one word covers an illness that comes in many forms and in various degrees; it causes the sufferer to feel agitated and anxious causing insomnia, feelings of worthlessness and guilt, and many more unpleasant symptoms. On the whole this leaves a low self-esteem and low self-worth.

A low self-esteem is a hugely common symptom of depression but can often be unrecognised or misdiagnosed. Many people who suffer with depression feel that they 'deserve' to feel the way they do, they do not think that others will be interested; they couldn't be further from the truth. No-one deserves to suffer with depression, people do care that their friends and loved ones are suffering. Just because those with depression have a low opinion of themselves it does not preclude them from other people's help.

Since the days of our ancestors we look back through time and appreciate how difficult life could be for them and we count ourselves lucky. How easy do we have it today? Years ago many people had very little in comparison to today and I would wager that there were fewer people suffering depression back then as there are now. I am not saying depression didn't exist then because it did. In today's Dot Com era we are not happy enough to keep up with the Jones' we are trying to keep up with The Jetsons' all craving the latest mobile phone, striving for the flattest and most enormous television in the street even if it means building an extension to house it. We run up massive credit card and store card debts to look like those on the covers of the glossy magazines. In order to achieve this we work longer and harder to pay off the credit cards, put fuel in our gas guzzling cars and pay the mortgage on houses that cripple the bank account. But we have never had it so easy.

"Pull Yourself Together"

Depression is something that touches us all, if it doesn't happen directly to you then it can certainly affect someone who is close to you. It can be triggered by a sudden lifestyle change or right of passage eg death, divorce and redundancy. It is an illness that affects the entire body, not just the mind, our mind is the computer which controls what we do, and therefore it can affect the body and soul too. The symptoms can be unpleasant, it can leave the person feeling in a constant negative state with a lack of vision for the bleak future, they can experience change in their weight with a lack of appetite and a lethargic state for which their body stops operating at full steam, they simply go through the motions of getting through the day. The opposite could happen too, some may carelessly comfort eat rich high fat foods that will cause them to gain weight rapidly.

The best cure is the good old fashioned saying "a problem shared is a problem halved". There are loved ones, friends and professionals that can help us through this difficult time, talking through and facing the problems can offer enlightening solutions. Medication can be prescribed such as antidepressants, and this medication when administered with counselling or coaching has been very effective in past cases. It is not an overnight remedy, it requires a lot of determination, it can feel like you have hit rock bottom, just remember from there, the only way is up!

Depression is not something you should be ashamed of nor is it an indication of personal weakness. It is something we may all experience. It is not a case of "pulling yourself together"; it's about working towards being an even stronger person than you were before.

Feeling that you are different from the rest of the world is the most uncomfortable feeling; you feel that you are the outsider looking into a not-so-perfect world but yearning to be a part of it regardless. It can leave you feeling physically, mentally and emotionally drained. A positive mental attitude seems light years away and it is far easier to bathe in negativity, where it is safe and comfortable after a while.

LIAH LAVASSUER'S STORY

"I knew I was bisexual since I was like seven or eight years old. It was strange feeling like that at such a young age. It's like you know something isn't right but you can't quite put your finger on it – does that make sense? Anyway, I always felt like there was more to me than the other little guys and girls.

I wasn't really bullied because of my sexuality; I know how to fight really well so people knew not to mess with me. I was scared when I came out, at first. Then after I adjusted along with everyone else I realised that I would rather have people in my life who liked me for me and not have to please others and feel torn up inside.

I came out first by telling my friend Tara, she's actually my first same sex relationship and I also put it on my profile page on FaceBook. I then came out at school, I received a mixed response, some girls thought it weird; and the rest didn't care one way or the other. Those who thought it weird thought they were a potential target but I had no interest in any of them, but if that's what they wanted to think I just let them think it. My first relationship came when I was about nine, it was with a guy but I was just following the crowd, in hindsight my first gay relationship came when I was fourteen, I think? I am pretty sure I was fourteen.

My coming out went better than I thought, luckily. Plenty of people saw it on their status updates and it spread like wild fire around some of my friends and acquaintances but on the whole I was relieved and I was being true to myself. My true colours were on full display for all to see. My friends have always been cool with it and society seems to be too.

When it came to telling my parents, let's just say I didn't get the response I was hoping for. I told my mom, she just replied "No you're not" and then casually walked away. What do you do after that happens? I sure didn't know.

184

Not long after I came out as being bi-sexual many of the girls and guys in my town started coming out as being bisexual. I think it became a bit of a trend because come a year later, almost all said they were just confused. It was just hilarious to witness but frustrating that they were taking something very real as being something to experiment with. One good thing came from this; it did open people's eyes towards those who are gay and bi-sexual. Now the people in my town are more accepting of gay rights than they were before.

I would have to say that coming out was almost the best thing I have ever done, if the response from my mom was more positive then it would have been great. She still loves me; it's just her way of dealing with it.

I am very in touch with my religious beliefs and believe that many people misunderstand The Holy Bible and interpret it for their own piece of mind. The gay people within The Bible didn't get punished for being gay, it was because they were choosing to be gay and raping people. I don't believe for one second that God doesn't like people that are gay, only if they choose to be disobedient.

I went to see a Counsellor from the age of twelve until I was fifteen. It was at a time when I was getting in touch with my true feelings and it took its toll, it required a lot of emotional and mental strength to discover the real me. I became sick and tired of going to my counselling sessions and by the time I made the decision to stop going things started to make sense and got a heck of a lot easier.

I believe that we are no different from those who are straight. We want to be loved, get married, some want kids and most people I meet just want to get through life happily and safely".

21 EASY Steps To Overcome Depression

If you believe that you are depressed then the first thing you need to do is speak to your doctor. Again, if you are offered medication and you believe you need it then work with them. Do not turn away the help that is being offered to you, use your own judgement and be sure to ask lots of questions. Take all the time you need. I know the time available with a doctor isn't that long but it is your health and that is important. That is why they are there.

Here are 21 easy steps that you can implement as well as any medication you might use.

1. DECIDE WHAT YOU WANT

The first thing you will need in order to succeed is a burning desire to overcome this thing called Depression. It is natural to want your old life back, but you will get more than that, you will get an even better life when you overcome it - honestly, it's true. Keep a journal, express your feelings and make positive goals for the future. As you achieve your goals you will see a vast difference in your attitude and your feelings.

2. WATCH WHAT YOU EAT / DRINK

There is a lot of truth in the age old saying – 'You will only get out, what you put in'. If you know categorically that your diet is no good then change it. The food you eat is reflected in your mood, your complexion, your health and your physique. You don't have to cut out everything and start from scratch. Have a look through a healthy eating cook book at your library or local book shop and then introduce the foods you need to have a healthy mind and healthy body. If you believe that you are deficient or require a boost of extra vitamins and minerals then go and visit your health food shop where these people know their stuff and enjoy nothing better than taking time to pass their knowledge onto you. The Vitamin B group are your brains best mates as without wanting to get too technical they grease the wheels of your mental functions. And as a footnote, drink plenty of water and as boring as it sounds, keep alcohol to moderation as it is a depressant.

3. WATCH WHAT YOU SAY

How many times have you called yourself stupid for forgetting to do something or for not knowing something? As innocent as it may seem you are talking to your subconscious – your 'inner self' if you will. By doing this you are breaking two major rules. Firstly you are telling yourself that you are stupid and secondly you are telling yourself that it is okay to be criticised. If it's not okay for me to call you stupid, then it's not okay for you to do it either. These words are a major contribution towards having negative and limiting beliefs. These are easily undone by taking the negative sentence and reversing it to the positive and repeat it and repeat it and repeat it until it is lodged firmly in your mind (remember the exercise in Chapter One). If you can't say anything nice, then do not say anything at all.

4. WATCH WHAT YOU... WATCH

It is very easy to sit down and watch those television programmes that allow us to switch off and require no thought at all. I am talking about daytime television here, particularly talk shows where you get the host, bringing out the first guest who is the injured party and then the perpetrator is brought on and then it all kicks off. It usually results in a lie detector test or DNA test being taken and then we wait for the results to be announced (I think we all know to whom we refer). I personally love these shows, I am a people watcher so I enjoy them purely for entertainment purposes; nevertheless they are no good for your mental health if you are in a depressed state. They are negative and quite toxic unless you are in a frame of mind where you can rise above the negativity. It is just as easy to change the channel and watch programs that send a different message or entertain through education. Steer clear of the movies that give you nightmares – watch light hearted stuff that makes you laugh and re-enforces the message that life is good. Watch things that are easy to follow and uplifting.

5. WATCH WHAT YOU READ

There are a lot of people that cannot pick up the newspaper without commenting and getting het up about the headlining stories. If this is you, then avoid them. If you feel that you need to keep up with the news or current affairs then limit how you receive the information. Perhaps watch the headlines at the top of the hour and then leave it at that. If you are just one of those people who love to read then make sure that you choose books that can help you with your development. There are some great self help books out there, improve those areas where you know you are lacking and brush up with them. I personally love reading the books and listening to the recordings of Napoleon Hill, he is such a joy to read and listen to. He carries a real firm message of the law of attraction and explains the importance of a positive mental attitude. Please visit **www.ClosetsAreForClothes.co.uk** where you can find out more about the inspirational works of Napoleon Hill.

6.   WATCH WHAT YOU LISTEN TOO

The greatest thing since sliced bread is the audio CD or MP3. You do not need to be alone when you are in the car or whilst you are walking to work, you can surely find your favourite book or favourite motivational speaker on CD or at the click of a button as a digital download, so use that time in the car or on foot to create a better frame of mind by listening to these recordings instead of the negative thoughts in your head. You may want to be selective about your music too, there is nothing better than listening to a song with a lot of feeling and emotion but do not bathe in this music, choose the music that gets you grabbing for the hairbrush and dancing around the living room. Be selective about who you are mixing with, keep those people who have a negative influence or demeanour at arms length, they maybe a close friend or loved one. Either explain that the negative things they are saying are not helping or just limit the time you see them. The most important person at this stage is you and you alone.

7.   IMMERSE YOURSELF IN FRIENDSHIP

Feelings of isolation are natural however you have friends and family who love and care for you. Use your time wisely, get out of the house and have a cup of tea with them, call them regularly for an update, especially those who live away. Catch up with those emails your friends have sent – the ones you have been meaning to do for so long. Now is as good a time as any. Arrange a weekly night out (it doesn't have to involve alcohol or large amounts of money) go to the cinema or arrange a takeaway night and take it in turns to host it. Keep all your lines of communication open so that you have a strong network of support. It is easy to shut yourself away – those who love you would rather be with you unwell, than not with you at all. Those are your real friends.

8. TALK... AND KEEP TALKING

Speak about your experiences or just talk through the way you are feeling, this is a simple but powerful therapy. The more you talk the more you will come to your own conclusions and find the right answers. Everything you need is within you; I will say that again: Everything you need is within you. It is just a case of finding it. Talking can be physically, emotionally and mentally draining. These symptoms happen for a reason and that is because once it is out, it has been acknowledged and it has been put to rest so you can fill the space with something positive.

9. GET OUT THERE

Sitting around the house is not the best use of your time. When you are down it is understandable that the urge to get ready and go out has vanished. Your enthusiasm and motivation are low and you would prefer not to see anyone. This really is no good for you, go for a walk or a run if that is something you used to enjoy. It is important to get out there and see some daylight, feel the warmth of the sun on your face, even the winter sun, the chill of the morning air and a deep breath can help.

10. POSITIVE ROUTINES

A lot of what we do becomes routine after a while; we carry out our duties most of the time unaware that we are doing them. It is important to lose the disruptive routines and make sure that you are implementing new and positive ones instead. One thing that many people fall short of doing is getting enough sleep. This is the best routine to get right: Go to bed at the same time every evening, have a hot bath/shower an hour before bed and listen to relaxing music or read a book. Getting a good night's sleep is a crucial factor in overcoming depression. Our conscious mind has to switch off.

11. EXERCISE – REBUILD YOUR TEMPLE

Exercise is a fantastic, low cost way to overcome depression. We have all had the gym membership that we have bought in the New Year; we go religiously in January only to give up in February. We see the standing order going out of the account every month and feel fitter just knowing we have paid the money. BIG MISTAKE! Take regular exercise, it helps you mentally to thrash out any negative feelings, you will see a noticeable change to your body and this will make you feel good, as well as looking great. The biggest motivation is seeing and feeling the results. So just start doing it and before long it will become as habitual as putting milk in your tea. It only needs to be 15 minutes a day, or every other day and you don't have to go to the gym. Why not join the local pool and swim, or buy an exercise DVD that features your favourite celebrity, or go for a long walk. Now for the science bit, many studies have been carried out and the conclusion is that physical exercise has a profound effect on the mind and soul. Exercising will significantly increase the levels of serotonin and dopamine in the brain which are the happy hormones.

12. THE THREE 'R's' – READING, 'RITING AND RELAXATION

There are so many creative activities that you can do that will mentally stimulate you and open a new world of infinite possibilities. Taking up a creative hobby can distract you from the things that make you unhappy. You may have a creative flair for writing, drawing, painting, music or fashion design. This can be healing and restorative, perhaps you are not skilled in any creative niche at present, so now might be a good time to attend an evening class to learn those skills you have always desired, or get a book on the subject and do it anyway. You might be highly skilled in reading out loud, there are websites that create and sell audio books, they might be looking for highly skilled readers to record their work. The point of introducing and encouraging a creative element to your life will offer relaxation and a positive form of expression.

190

13. MUSIC

Have you ever noticed that those movies that you watch from behind the sofa are never that scary when you press the mute button? Music can enhance or sour the mood and it has been proven that different types of music cause different reactions within the body. Classical music is great for increasing concentration and it is also used to relax and switch off. Upbeat music, especially those songs that take you back to a specific time that was happy and fun will soon have you smiling and thinking of happier times. Likewise, listening to music from unhappy times will have the undesired effect.

14. BE FORGIVING

Sometimes we might experience bad situations. Many things happen to us and we can end up disliking ourselves or others, or both. You may dislike yourself for causing a situation and regret having done it, perhaps someone has hurt you or been unkind and for that you can never forgive them, and you could then dislike yourself in return for letting them do that to you. Sound familiar? Be forgiving of yourself and others, you don't have to make huge gestures for this to work. If you have hurt someone in the past and you have lost contact and it haunts you, then just think about what you have done, hold the feeling, tell yourself that you forgive yourself and you will never do it again. Then release the feeling and push it away. The same will work for those who have hurt you and never apologised, they may be sorry now but for whatever reason can't or wouldn't say sorry.

15. BE GRATEFUL

The most powerful exercise that you can do is keep a journal each evening before going to bed write five things that you like about yourself and five things that you are thankful for. Counting your blessings sounds simple, but is effective. Write them down – see it literally. The best way to prevent repeating your entries is to look at that particular day for your inspiration – perhaps use your diary. As time goes by you will look at everything you do and everyone you meet as a reason to see the good. It is true that points make prizes. "What do points make…?"

16. RIDE OUT BAD THOUGHTS

When you think bad thoughts, it doesn't mean you are a bad person. It is easy to think you are going mad or losing the plot and you will be glad to hear that you are not mad. You are not losing the plot and you are not a bad person. Bad thoughts creep into our heads; these can be caused from the millions of messages that enter our brain on a daily basis, we sift through them, distort, delete or file them away for later. When we are fit and well we have the ability to ignore them, when we are depressed these thoughts bellow out in our head.

The best way to combat these is to not be afraid of them. Believe me when I say that it is your inner fear that keeps them alive and turns the volume up to the maximum.

The Stop! Technique might assist here as it is frequently used in cognitive-behavioural therapy. Therapists usually advise and teach this technique to clients in order to stop negative thoughts or compulsive worrying. This is something that you could do quite easily when you begin to feel any anxiety or pressure that is affecting your thoughts.

This technique is highly effective when the compulsive or negative thoughts begin. When you begin to feel these happen, shout clearly the word, "Stop!" This will allow you to replace it with a new and healthier thought pattern, just think of the things that make you happy like raindrops on roses and whiskers on kittens – that type of thing.

The reason that the Stop! Technique has been highly successful is because when you first shout out the word "Stop!" it helps focus the attention on the word which draws your attention away from the unhealthy thought. As you become accustom to doing this, in time you will be able to mentally shout the word without needing to say it out loud.

There are many techniques like this available, it is just a matter of browsing the internet or reading the correct books that have been written to improve positive thought patterns and eradicate negative behaviour.

As an alternative, you could try the Picture Power exercise in Chapter Twelve.

17. TAKING CONTROL

Always look forward and never look back. The past can hold some wonderful memories that you will remember and cherish forever. It also has incidents and occasions that you would rather forget – let them go. Every time you think of those memories you would rather not think about, replace them with a memory that you like, eventually your mind will replace the negative feelings with the positive image. *If you always do what you have always done, then you will always get what you have always got.* Don't be surprised that you are getting the same old results if you have not done anything to change them; it is only when you implement change that you will see things happen.

18. HAVE 'YOU' TIME

There are so many demands made on your time that it is important to be a little selfish on occasion and do the things you want to do. It is crucial for the sake of your mental health that you have 'me time' even if it is once a week. This can come in the form of reading a book whilst having a hot soak in the bath, going for a bit of retail therapy or booking a table for one at your favourite restaurant and having a date with yourself. Do whatever you want to do. I know plenty of people, all of whom are very popular who go to the cinema alone, or just do things in order to enjoy their own company. Personally, I am a lonesome shopper and prefer it. Be kind to yourself, bathe, buy nice bath salts and body cream – treat yourself.

Meditation is a great way to relax. Many are put off by meditation as they believe that it forms parts of other religious traditions that do not belong to their own, or there are special skills required to practice it. If that's the case don't call it meditation call it 'Me Time', switch the lights off, light a few candles or even do it the other way around to avoid an accident and put on your favourite chill-out music and just breathe slowly. That's all it is, that's meditation.

19. GET A COACH OR MENTOR

Unresolved problems with the past can be put to rest using the service of a Counsellor. Many respected practices will offer a free no-obligation consultation in order to establish whether or not they can assist, or refer you to a specialist professional that can best deal with your individual circumstances. This also allows you to see if you want to work with them in moving forward, you may meet or speak to them and decide that their service is not for you. Enrolling the assistance of a professional does not mean that you are defeated or even weak, quite the contrary: You are showing that you are strong, you have identified that there is something that requires work and you are doing something about it. Professional life coaches will also offer a free consultation and for the same reason you should use this to make your decision. Life coaching will primarily look towards the future. Your destiny is yours to create. Life coaching does allow you to look at the past in order to utilise tools that have helped you before and it is also good to look back to see exactly how far you have come.

20. GET AWAY

It doesn't have to be a lavish holiday, book a break away that is well within your budget and it doesn't have to be abroad. We take for granted all the wonderful places we have around us, so book a hotel, pack a bag and just retreat somewhere. Some time away from home and out of the normal routine of daily life can allow you to see the changes that are required to move forward. Give yourself something to look forward to, take the time to relax and work through your thoughts for that positive outcome.

A healthy body and healthy mind are crucial for a happy life. By implementing the other twenty points you will clear out the old and introduce the new. You can say goodbye to negativity and misery and say hello to positivity, peace and happiness. It is important to look at what you are doing, and find better ways to improve your quality of life. Detox doesn't have to be about drinking wheat grass for the rest of your days; it is about listening to your body and acting on it. We are told to drink more water, less caffeine and alcohol. Although many people raise the point that their tea or coffee contains water, so that contributes to the daily intake, you must remember that tea and coffee are diuretics which dehydrate the body.

Green tea is far better and full of antioxidants which have restorative benefits that protect and strengthen the body, the plain variety might not be to everyone's taste, so try a flavoured green tea – they are just as good for you.

Treating yourself to a massage could benefit your mind and body. A massage affects the nerve endings in the skin, like exercise this will release the happy hormones and will reduce your stress levels. Massages can lower blood pressure and increase the circulation of the blood too. Do a little research about the types of service in your area, go along and have a chat with a professional.

Colonic Hydrotherapy or Irrigation is not for everyone. This is where an infusion of warm filtered water is gently introduced under a low pressure into the colon; this removes a build up of waste and toxins from the body. If your body is not sufficiently hydrated then some water may get absorbed, this will help make skin look younger and fresh, it will also help with smoothing out those fine lines. This procedure may not be for everyone, and is probably not recommended during the period of depression, once you are safely over the depression this is something that might be of interest.

A Journey

Depression is a journey, albeit not a very pleasant one, as someone who has been there I can say in all honesty that there is life during and after depression. You will actually become stronger for having been through it, you will have to do so much soul searching to get through the other end, you feel the relief of having just completed a tough exam. In this exam you will mark the paper and you will feel the sheer relief and happiness when you have passed. There are many self help books out there; you can find them for sale online or in your local book shop.

Please visit **www.ClosetsAreForClothes.co.uk** as this contains resources that will assist you with this.

CHRISTOPHER BRANDON'S STORY

"I realised that I was gay when I was around eight years old. At that age my mother hadn't talked to me about sex education but I felt that what I was feeling was wrong in some way. Wrong meaning that it was socially unacceptable but it felt completely right in my heart.

I was bullied at school and by "friends". Girls would beat me up; I was tormented from Grade School through my sophomore year in High School.

Coming out was both traumatic and liberating at the same time. The whole family issue was the traumatic part. Coming out was liberating in the fact that I no longer had to live a life full of lies. That life of lies which contributed to much of my alcoholism.

I had my first gay relationship when I was eighteen. I was outed by circumstance. My stepfather had come to my apartment to get me for work when I pulled up with my boyfriend at the time on his motorcycle. My stepfather put two and two together and I was now out.

My "outing" experience was better than I had anticipated. Being outted, takes out the whole "what kind of speech am I going to give and to whom" process.

I have a terrific relationship with my parents, since coming out I have since found out that my biological father is gay. My stepfather is very accepting of my homosexuality. My mother is encouraging me to find a partner. We are even starting to compare notes about who we think are the most handsome male celebrities.

Before I came out I never thought it possible that I could have this support from friends and family, and now I can be myself I can truly say that it is THE best thing I have ever done in my life. Now I can live my life. Freely!

I suffered mentally because of my sexuality. I attempted suicide twice before coming out. Being in the closet for so many years led me down the road of alcohol and drug addiction. I came out twenty years ago. Today I remain alcohol free for three years and drug free for fourteen years. By accepting who I was as a person, ignoring what society says is "morally right" helped me to release a lot of the anger and resentment I held onto for so many years. Although I tried to live the life of a straight man I knew what I was, I never married a female however after having three heterosexual relationships I concluded that my true happiness was in a gay relationship.

I wish that there were more places for the GLBT community to meet on a regular basis. It is discouraging to think that in 2010 that we can only really be ourselves or to find a potential partner hidden in a bar scene or the classified ads".

Suicide

Suicide is a permanent solution to a very temporary problem. When you experience thoughts of suicide it usually means that you have reached rock bottom. These thoughts can seem like some type of comfort during a crisis, an easy way out but easy for whom. The end of life is a sad and dismal thing, but when it is ended through suicide it is far more of a waste – it seems even more heartbreaking because if all those close knew of the turmoil, then they would surely have helped.

Many people I have spoken to have thought about suicide as an easy way out – and not all of them were gay. For someone who is battling with their sexuality, death seems so much easier than actually telling loved ones those immortal words "I am gay". There are stories within these pages of real people who mention suicide as a remedy; I myself have experienced the dark thoughts of suicide. The first time during my schooldays, it seemed like a better solution than to go in day after day being verbally battered by those who thought they were better than me. If you think that I or anyone else might not understand, then I can tell you that we do. It's not something many people talk about, it's seen as a weakness to say you have thought of suicide, but it's not. It takes great strength to look suicide in the face and walk away, and continue living and just being yourself. I haven't told many people about wanting to take my own life but I am not ashamed, because I got through it. I am here as 'living' proof, I got through it and I am very, very happy to be here.

What stopped me from going through with it? I prayed for happier times, I prayed for strength and I imagined my mam and dad at my funeral, following my coffin, my aunties and uncles and how they would feel. I thought that just because my life wasn't that great, I wasn't going to destroy all their lives. Suicide is selfish because we seldom think of the people we leave behind. Yeah sure, our pain and suffering ends, but for them it has only just begun. In fact we feel nothing ever again. The warm sun on your face, the gentle breeze that gives you a shiver up your spine, the non-stop laughter over the silliest joke, the fuzziness inside from seeing someone you love smile. Yes, suicide really is that final, a little too final.

If you are feeling that suicide is the only remedy then you are at rock bottom. When you reach rock bottom you have a choice either sink or swim. To someone that doesn't understand it's like trying to explain the unexplainable, but when you have reached it... you will know. How? I don't know, but you will know. From there you can only go up and when those thoughts pass... and yes they do pass, you will be very glad you are still here.

The thing with suicide is that I don't think we really want to end it, we want to be caught or found in the nick of time and then this cry for help will be heard and things might change. Often we are not caught or found, and it might just be too late. The cry for help is not heard and another life is over, but could have been saved if someone knew what was really going on inside.

The wonderful thing about the human mind is it's there to protect, it's not self destructive, it is all powerful. There is always doubt; it's caused by the human mind as a safety function. Whilst the doubt emerges, strength is required to listen.

Thoughts of suicide does not mean you are going mad, are weak or even bad, it doesn't even mean that you want to die, but you just want an instant solution for your pain. It means that the pain, not a physical pain but the inner anguish, is so bad that you feel compelled to end it all. You feel that weighing up the options that the world will be a far better place without you in it. But, you are wrong; you are only seeing one half of the argument, all the negatives, the bad things. Just imagine for one moment that your friend came to you with the same negative emotions you are feeling, how would you correct them? You'd tell them how much you loved having them around, just being there, someone to talk to, to share moments with, to laugh with. You'd think about every funny little quirk of the character that makes them special in your eyes. If you can do that for them, why can't you do that for yourself? You really aren't all that different.

Remember that you are not the only one to feel like this, most of those that have, did not go through with it... unlike being gay; it is a passing phase because your mind and body want you to find the strength to get through it.

You can change how you feel and see yourself in an instant. You have the power within you to make the decision to live a happy and fulfilling life. There are many who have trod the dark boards of depression before you, but come out the other side and live extremely happy lives. Immerse yourself in good and positive things and be with positive and caring people. Watch your favourite comedies over and over, the ones that make you laugh every time, despite knowing what's coming. Arrange to meet up with the people you enjoy spending time with, just be around happy and positive influences.

Headaches are normally treated with painkillers but there is only one cure for the pain of inner turmoil. It is perseverance with a positive mental attitude. Remember that today is tomorrow's yesterday. The negative present moment doesn't have to be your future; it can be your past. Tomorrow is another day and it will get easier until you find happiness again. You were happy and content before feeling suicidal therefore happiness will come again, it might need perseverance – there's that word again, but it will be fine.

Suicide has a stigma about it, because it is a part of death people feel uneasy about it. Death is negative, it has never been seen as a good thing because is causes pain, heartache and black voids in the lives of others. Talking to someone whether a loved one, a friend, a person you trust or a professional such as your Doctor, a Counsellor, a Psychotherapist, a Life Coach – anyone who has a caring nature, an ear to listen and someone who has your best interests at heart. They will not think you are crazy, they will just know you are experiencing huge amounts of pain. You will not be burdening anyone with your pain; you will just be borrowing strength until yours is running at maximum capacity.

Talk with someone about your feelings and keep them regularly updated. They will care about you, it can be over the phone but it is far better to do it one to one with a cup of tea or coffee. If you don't want to be on your own then don't be. Ask your friends or family for support you need to make you happy and strong and I'm sure they will not think twice about giving it.

Mix and spend time with positive people. You know the ones, those who have a laugh and enjoy life, not the dreary type who always see the bad side of life. Spend time with those who make you happy and spend time doing activities that make you smile.

Remove any objects from the house that you have perhaps thought of as an aid to suicide. This can be medication, sharp or dangerous objects. They will be a reminder to you; get rid of them until you know that you can have them safely in your home.

Finally, by following the 21 step programme in this chapter it will allow you to clear your mind, body and soul of anything that is unwanted.

Self Harming

People self harming for many different reasons, usually because of a painful or traumatic period experienced in youth. With nowhere to turn, it's an emotional release. It is used when a person's emotional pain is so unbearable they cause themselves physical pain to counteract it. Some self harm is carried out as a form of punishment, others as a form of control, and some do it as a reminder that they are alive.

It can come in many forms such as hair pulling, burning or cutting the flesh, punching walls (until they bleed), nail biting, alcohol or drug abuse. Anorexia and Bulimia are also forms of self-harm, purposely depriving the body of food as a method of showing control and causing damage and destruction.

If you self harm then you are not alone, you are not crazy, mad, or a bad person. It is however a sign that you feel powerless or insecure, you do not love yourself as you feel you should. The first thing you need to do is decide that you do love and care for yourself, that you are worthy of a perfect body, free from the harm and damage that you have inflicted. You must make the conscious decision that you do not want to self harm any longer and take steps to move away from this. There is a reason you began harming yourself, it boils down to one of your life's significant events.

Depression and frustration are usually the feelings felt by the person who wishes to cause themselves harm. Remember to confide in those who care for you, talking is the answer. Do not let everything build up inside, this isn't good for you.

Once you have decided that you wish to overcome it then you need to speak to someone. A visit to the Doctor, which is always 100 per cent confidential, will help guide you in the right direction. Remember, you have the information super highway at your fingertips so have a look online for organisations and advice as this might be helpful.

A great way of forgetting your troubles, and the self harming, is to do the things you enjoy. The 21 step programme in this chapter will allow you to break bad habits and also offer positive distraction. It's about being happy, supported by those who care for you and dealing with life's problems so they don't result in physical injury.

Keep doing the things that make you happy and once you begin to break the pattern, you will feel much better. If it doesn't work then you really do need to speak to someone. Whoever you tell will care and will want to help because if they care for you, they will only have your best interests at heart.

The best thing to do is see your Doctor. Just think they have seen it all before (probably much worse) so don't think they will judge you in any way. They are there to help, you may not recognise this, but if they didn't want to help, they would have chosen a different profession.

I will finish by saying that you need to take care. Continuous harm to the flesh can result in permanent scarring or serious infection. If you have a wound that doesn't look right or is not healing then see your Doctor.

Social Networking Site Warning:

Spending too much time online can have an impact on your mental state leaving you feeling depressed. There is now an epidemic of internet addicts who are hooked on surfing the information super highway, and social networking and dating websites are a major cause of this. These sites are beginning to replace conventional interaction.

Like any addiction it can consume a person's concentration from the important responsibilities of everyday life such as performance at work and interfering with the smooth running of the home when chores are being discarded for the next internet fix. Although the amount of time spent on the internet is an indication of a person's addiction, it is more to do with the subject's relationship with the internet. It is crucial to limit internet use and realise the importance of interacting with people in the way nature intended. Can you remember the days before mobile phones? No, me neither.

CHAPTER FOURTEEN

A Word To Parents, Siblings, Relatives, Friends And Those On Your Christmas Card List

It can be difficult for those who are coming to terms with having a gay child, relative or friend. I am sure that it's not an ideal situation for you when someone you love drops the bombshell and tells you that they are gay. You thought that you knew them inside and out, and now begin to question whether you really knew them at all. In fact, you did know them very well and still do, however now you will have much more enjoyment with them as they become a much improved person, with heightened confidence and self-esteem, with a reassurance of self-worth and feel comfortable for being accepted for their true feelings. It is understandable if you feel like a small bomb has gone off, if you had no idea that they had been fighting with themselves about their feelings of difference. But now that you are aware of their true feelings, you will have a better understanding.

Most parents will experience emotions of anger, denial, sadness, worry, confusion – primarily thinking about what they must have gone through when they needed to talk and how they did not know. You may also be expressing emotions and feel the pain that you will not see your child settle down in the way you had always imagined. This is a difficult time for you, however, without wanting to sound harsh – this is not about *you*. It is about the person you love and care about, the one who has just taken the biggest step in their life by sharing something that they thought they would have to keep hidden forever.

There are so many parents out there who want to give the best help and support to their child. I have been approached by many parents, mainly mothers, who say that they suspect their child might be gay. It is great that some parents can perhaps recognise the early signs so they can be on hand at the crucial moment to show their child that it's okay to be the person they really want to be. When does that crucial moment come? Who knows, it happens when it happens, when the time is right one way or another.

CALSEY TURNER'S STORY

"I have known my whole life that I was gay, I have always been more attracted to women and like most people I tried to hide it and even deny it to myself. I came to terms with it when I was fifteen years old, I was lucky to have a friend who helped me through the whole process of acknowledging it for myself.

When I came out to my friends on my softball team I started to get bullied and teased for being myself. They told their parents who then started attacking me because they didn't want me to "hit on their daughters". At school, I was lucky and I didn't experience much bullying. There were a few closed minded kids who would make hurtful and spiteful remarks, but for the most part everyone was okay with it. I experienced two responses, there were those who supported me and accepted it and there were those who didn't say anything about it.

When I decided to come out, I had never been so nervous in my life. I had been with my girlfriend for seven months. My mom decided to look through my text messages and saw the ones from her and flipped out. She started screaming and hitting me telling me I was a disgrace to the family and that I was not her daughter anymore. I ran away that day, I was seventeen years old and I vanished for three days. My father was of little help as he has been very religious since a small child.

I am not out to all of my extended family yet. I want to tell them but feel like I can't because my mom has planted it in my head that I am a disgrace to the family and I can't let anyone else know or they will all hate me too. I know deep down that some of my family will accept me; I am just afraid that they may react in the same way as my parents. I knew my parents would need some time to get used to it but I never thought they would disown me. It is a horrible feeling but at the same time I feel accomplished. In the beginning I wanted to take it all back and say it was just a phase but I knew it would only get worse if they ever saw me with my girlfriend, and it did. I had wanted to tell them for a while at that point but I didn't know how to broach the subject. Since it just happened all at once it was over and done before I knew it, it took its own course. It was as if a huge weight had been lifted even if they did take it badly. I no longer have to hide or pretend I am something I am not.

It disheartens me a bit when I think that my relationship with my friends is the same since coming out, they still see me as the same person I was before but my mom hates me even though she says she accepts me now. She never talks to me about anything anymore like we used to, she wont dare mention anything about my life and what I'm doing, she doesn't want anything to do with me anymore. The only reason I can't move out and get a place of my own is because she wants to know where I am at all times and who I am hanging out with.

I cannot be sure if it has been the best thing I have ever done or the worst. Where I have gained in one aspect I have lost out in another. I want to say it's the best, because it set me free from the chains established by my parents and by society. However, it is one of the worst, because it destroyed the relationship I had with them. Overall, I would say it was better than not telling them.

When I came out I had to drop my faith and religious beliefs. It was not through choice but I was banned from all the churches in my area. I concluded that if God could forgive a child molester or murderer and not me because of whom I choose to love, I would not believe anymore as I'm going to burn in hell anyway, right?

I have battled mentally with the whole saga of coming out and being gay. I am not sure if this chain of events was caused by my sexuality or because I came out − perhaps a mixture of the two. I became very depressed and attempted to take my own life by overdosing on pain killers. I became addicted to Tylenol with codeine and other powerful over the counter drugs. My friends found out when I dropped my pills one day, it was then they sat me down and told me how much I meant to them and the impact I had on all their lives, and how I needed to be alive to really enjoy all the small things in life.

My friends have truly been my saving grace. I have a good circle of friends on and off the gay scene. The gay scene is something I love, the public's view of it, however, I do not. Our community is perceived as a sex driven crowd of nonconformists who will screw anything as long as it has legs and a pulse. The media has not helped, I feel they have given the gay community a bad reputation and I believe that is why we are not accepted amongst the general public".

Here are a few things you might want to consider while you are supporting the one you love as they have just told you that they are gay.

No Fuss

There is no need for a fuss, stay calm and collected. They are no different to the person they were five minutes ago – before they told you they were gay. They are not unwell and do not require anything other than understanding. At this point it's you that is in shock, they have had years and years to get used to this so at this point they will feel vulnerable. At the same time they will feel as light as a feather having had a huge weight lifted from their shoulders. Carry on as normal, just do the things you do everyday; they are not a 'special case' and they require no special treatment. It will be enough just to reassure them and show them that you love them and that nothing will change. Tell them that you love them too; this is what they will want to hear – business as usual.

Coming To Terms

As a parent you may feel that you have failed in your duty because your son/daughter has told you that they are gay. This is categorically not the case. Some parents may even feel that their child has failed them for being gay, but there is no blame here. No-one is at fault as there is not one thing that anyone could have done to make an alternative outcome.

I remember telling my dad, who was extremely understanding about my being gay, that he was no less of a man for having a gay son. He knew that, and his response was "I know that" and he meant it. In fact, the way he handled it showed him to be the amazing person I know he is. He could have reacted in so many different ways, and as my dad; he reacted the way I would have expected. It saddens me when I think of others who are in the same position who get the opposite response from their parents.

You only fail your child if you are not there for them when they face a difficult dilemma – even if it's something you cannot help with or influence. The fact of the matter is, as long as you are there for them when times get tough, you are living up to your responsibilities.

This is also a period of change for you as well as them so take time to come to terms with it and keep all levels of communication open.

Don't Attach A Label

When you speak about your child then make sure you hold them in the same esteem as you did before. You don't have to tell the world by renaming them 'my gay son' or 'my gay daughter'. If it comes up in conversation and you feel you want a person to know then do it. You wouldn't have to tell people that your child is straight so there is no need to tell people that they are gay. Take care who you tell, for your sake more than anything else. The reason I say this is because if someone looks surprised or perhaps does not agree with homosexuality they might make it clear and being the parent, your protective side may just emerge.

"You'll Grow Out Of It"

It is easy for your first response to be either "Are you sure?", "It's a phase" or "You'll grow out of it". These three responses do not assist in making the situation better; this will just block the levels of communication. There have been many people who have told their parents that they are bi-sexual when they are in actual fact gay. They do this because is does not seem as severe as being told that they are gay and it also allows some glimmer of hope that they might end up in a straight relationship. It's buying time really.

If your child tells you that they are bi-sexual then take it with the same calm and collected attitude and allow them to explore themselves as a person. They might be bi-sexual and therefore might be looking for the right partner regardless of gender.

I was about seven years old when I knew I was different to everyone else. I might have actually been younger, and once I had entered the realms of puberty I realised that I had no attraction towards girls. Be aware that your child is not too young to know how they feel; they will not know what it is that makes them different, but they *do* know that they are different from their friends and classmates.

Unlimited Hugs, Kisses And Understanding

Be on hand to give them a hug and a kiss when they need it or however you usually reassure them. Be there to listen when they need to speak and hand them a tissue when they get upset. That's all they really want and be sure to tell them it will be alright and give them whatever they need so they can get used to their new start. You are still their parent, the person they seek comfort from.

When it comes to understanding, you may not have met another gay person before so it can be difficult to deal with this as you have no one to turn to who might understand. This is why I hope this book is beneficial to you. My advice to you is to do what comes naturally, read this book to get an idea of what's to come so you can work through it with them as opposed to them going it alone. My parents didn't know any gay people when I came out and thinking about it they don't know any now apart from those I have introduced them to.

HANNAH DAVENPORT'S STORY

"I began wondering if I liked girls when I was about fourteen years old. Only now have I realised that I truly am gay, before this it was like a type of 'limbo' where I wondered if I was gay perhaps bi, I'm not sure.

I know I am lucky when I say that I have never been bullied by anyone at school, I didn't come out until after High School so I didn't go through the torture of the other kids knowing and making my life hell because of it, and I'm careful who I tell, even today. This might be due to the fact I have a cousin who is very conservative, they like to make snide remarks about 'dykes' or 'lesbos' whenever I'm around. Yes it hurts; especially when these remarks come from one of your own family. You would expect it from someone outside the family, from someone who doesn't feel duty bound to love or care for you, but I would never have expected it from flesh and blood

My coming out was probably a little different to most, although most of the people I meet all have a different story to tell. My parents found out about my sexuality through my cousin, so it was pretty terrifying because I had no control over it. I was attending college at the time, my cousin saw my MySpace page, which said that I was bi-sexual, and told my mom, who then immediately called me and said that we needed to talk. To cut a long story short it was an awful experience. My mom and I cried, and I felt so guilty and dirty, like I had committed some kind of crime. Afterwards it felt like the weight had become heavier rather than lighter as most people describe it. I felt bad, and I was upset, because I didn't think any of my family would find out. Perhaps it would have been different if I had taken control of the situation but I didn't think my cousin would out me. I didn't give it a thought.

It is only now that my relationship with my parents is starting to level out. We didn't have the greatest relationship before my coming out, so

211

it's hard to tell. One thing is for sure, it's such a relief to be myself, with my family members that know, and all my friends.

It was both the best thing I had ever done and the worst. If I could go back and do it over, I would wait until I was more independent, at least before telling my parents. I like being different, and I hated having to hide that, I like being myself too.

I do feel that I am suffering with an internal battle because my faith doesn't understand my feelings. How often? Oh, every day. Only in the past year have I come to grips with my own lack of belief in an organised religion. It's a terrible feeling to know that some of my family worry, thinking I'm going to burn forever in hell for being gay.

My first real relationship came when I was nineteen years old, it was with a woman and she was nine years my senior.

I did have a few mental health issues the year I was outed. I withdrew from college and moved back in with my parents, and my mom would say things like "I don't know if I want you to take a bath in my tub because you might have AIDS". She really made me feel like the scum of the earth, which she had a knack for anyway. It's a hard feeling to describe, but it's like you're the most horrible worthless person alive, almost like I was a murderer or rapist or something. I guess the main things that helped me through times like that was my GSA group from college, and my great-aunt, who always treated me the same, no matter what she knew or heard about me.

Like most people I went to find solace in the gay scene but if I am honest I think there is a lot of drama to be found there, as far as dating goes. Don't get me wrong it is great for getting out, meeting new people, having some drinks - and dancing. But it's not likely that you're going to find a meaningful relationship there. I have been involved in arguments on multiple occasions on the scene with this girl I liked, once because a 'friend' of mine told her I was hitting on some girl she liked, and another time because she was making stupid life decisions and I was scared for her.

At the moment I am single and just enjoy being me".

Always The Bridesmaid, Never The Bride

When your child comes into the world you very quickly move from helping them with their first steps to imagining what their lives will be like when they become young adults. You will want them to get the best education possible, perhaps go to University, get a great job and find that special someone to walk with them down the aisle. As you tick these things off the list you are told that your vision of their future is going to change a little because they are attracted to the same sex.

After the initial shock of your child telling you their real feelings you will become closer. As time moves on as you appreciate the journey they have made.

As parents you will only want the absolute best for your child. You will want them to be well mannered and respectful of others. Many parents at the point of being told their child is gay have gone into complete meltdown. They believe that life as they know it is over and that is that. On the other hand many parents remain calm and collected and offer love and support from the start. By keeping all lines of communication open, you will become happier and closer.

Many parents, particularly mothers, may miss the big white wedding; a father might feel the void of not giving his daughter away on the biggest day of her life. Thankfully gay partnerships are now recognised and celebrated so you can see your son or daughter take to the aisle and marry the one he or she loves, should they and their partner wish to. Again, they may wish to have children in order to create a happy and stable family. These children may not be biologically your grandchildren but there are so many children in this world that need love and if your son or daughter decide to create a family through adopting they will still be your family.

You may need to prepare yourself for the fact that your son or daughter might not want to tie the knot or have children. In actual fact this might have happened were they born heterosexual. We are not all cut out for marriage or to be parents.

If You Think Your Child Might Be Gay

If you suspect that your son or daughter is gay and they haven't approached you then your feelings of concern and anxiety are natural. The best advice in order to make the whole situation a little easier, is by explaining to them that when people grow up, that men find love with women and vice versa and a man can also find love with another man and women can find love with another woman. Reassure them that it is not wrong to be attracted to people of the same sex.

You only have one life, it's not a dress rehearsal, so make it a happy one with the time you have got. No matter if your child is gay, straight or a hairdresser, just love them for who they are.

I sincerely wish you the best of luck.

CHRISTOPH STEFFEN'S STORY

"I'm twenty-six now and fully at peace with who I am. It hasn't always been as plain sailing as this though. When I was about twelve or thirteen years old I realised that I was attracted to men, and this was confirmed when I was sixteen years old and I was attracted to a really cute guy. I was never "out" at school but everyone seemed to know about my sexuality, it was as if they could tell. I spent a lot of my school years in fear because my classmates and other pupils would make fun of me and be quite cruel. It's not a time I look back on fondly.

To say it was easy suppressing my feelings deep inside and pretending to be something I wasn't was not easy at all. You feel like you want nothing more than to come out but there are so many reasons why it is a good idea to say nothing and carry on. I knew I should do it but was afraid to lose people, and be judged by all those who knew me. It affected my very being, I could not escape it even to the point that I couldn't sleep because of all this stuff in my head.

214

I decided to come out and the only way I could do it was by sending my best friend a text message from my mobile phone to hers. I knew she had other gay friends so she might understand and be sympathetic. As I suspected all went well and then I decided to send a letter to my mother while I was doing my military service. I am sad to say that it didn't go that well as my mother is a devout Catholic; she questioned many things like what she had done wrong and was it because my father died when I was young. It was upsetting to watch my mother question herself, however I felt free as well. It was like I could scream into the world: HELLO EVERYONE IM GAY!

Since that day it wasn't a problem for my brother or stepfather, but my mother reacted differently. At first it was hell, I sent her letter after letter whilst on service away and nothing. When I came back, she didn't talk to me for a long while and that was the most hurtful thing of all, because we lived in the same flat. I was at my wits end, my self-esteem was at my lowest because my mother was completely ignoring me.

It was the best thing I had ever done but it came at a price of hurting my mother, but it hurt me more, I was unable to be who I was. Since coming out I am far more outgoing, I was really very shy before and the only way I could deal with the situation was to self harm. I used to cut my arms in order to deal with my inner turmoil but this has stopped and I am happy with life.

I would visit the scene very occasionally just to meet up with others who understood my background and where I was coming from. I had some good nights but it was important to take care as there were a lot of drugs being handed out, it is important to look after your personal safety when you are out. I only ever had one bad experience and that was during my very first night on the scene. This older guy approached me and began undoing my shirt, not being that familiar with the scene and also being a little shocked I didn't know what to do. My friend could see I was being taken advantage of, she basically said that his death would be the only outcome if he didn't stop touching me. I would never go on the scene alone, only with friends.

I am happier today than I ever thought possible. They say time is a great healer, because now my mother is the complete opposite to how she was. It was only last week when our immediate family went to a restaurant for a meal – my boyfriend was invited and was sat with my brother and I. Whilst there she met an old friend who asked "Are these your sons?" My mother replied "No, just these two, and this is my eldest son's boyfriend". I was so proud! It was then I knew she had accepted my boyfriend, and more importantly accepted me. Who knows what the future will hold, perhaps marriage, but we have a lot of living to do first and we have to decide which one of us is going to wear the wedding dress. I'm joking!"

CHAPTER FIFTEEN

Transgender

This topic could be written in a book of its own. My reason for incorporating it into this book is simply to educate those who are unsure of what the term, *transgender*, really means. I hope I am able to assist in your understanding the individuals who put 'T' in LGBT.

The word transgender is a general term given to a variety of individuals or groups of individuals who challenge the gender role given to them at birth.

Those who are transgender begin life with the body they are born with, they find that they are extremely unhappy with what has been assigned to them through nature and then make the brave decision to undergo the necessary changes to make them happy. This is done through prescribed hormones, plastic surgery and electrolysis.

What's The Difference Between A Lesbian, Gay, Bi-sexual And Transgender Individual?

The difference is this, whether you are straight, gay, lesbian or bi-sexual we are pretty much comfortable with our own sexuality and gender. Those who are transgender are perhaps comfortable with their sexuality but not with their gender. Many people who have had issues with their gender have often said "I was a woman trapped in man's body" or "I was a man trapped in a woman's body". It must be difficult because to them they think, feel and do everything as a woman would but their gender says otherwise. Those who are transgender don't necessarily identify with being straight, gay, lesbian, bi-sexual or asexual on the basis that it poses the question 'Is a post-op female-to-male transsexual who finds love with another man gay?' and vice versa.

It would seem that there is a deep rooted sense of shame embedded within those who know they were born different because of sexuality, gender or any other differences that society do not deem 'normal'. This shame is similar to the feelings a gay, lesbian or bi-sexual person might have about their sexuality. Initially we fight what we feel in a desperate attempt to fit in and be accepted by our friends, family, colleagues and just the average person walking down the street. It is harder for a transgender person to hide themselves, after they have made the leap to change what they didn't like over those hiding their sexuality. It is as if those struggling with their sexuality are battling with the inside but those who are struggling with their gender are battling with their outside – but that battle takes place on the inside too.

The usual procedure to assist those who wish to make the change to become the person they have always wanted to be, usually begins with counselling and then down the line prescribed courses of hormones to assist with the change, then eventually surgery.

Opinions on transgender issues have opened up theories that there is an overlapping in identities in the categories of transsexuals, transvestites, cross-dressers and drag queens. We will go a little further into detail with these groups later on.

Before we continue, you may be wondering what the difference between transgender and transsexuals are. The easiest way to explain this is that transgender is an umbrella term that refers to anyone whose behaviours, thoughts, feelings or human traits differ from society's expectations of their assigned gender.

In conclusion, transgender means the group as a whole, it would seem that they are lumped together yet they are all different and we will look at each individual sub group e.g. transsexual, crossdresser and transvestite. We also look at female impersonator or drag queens as they are more commonly known as they are often misinterpreted as being a form of transgender. Here we will look at them individually.

Transsexual persons identify and have a longing to be accepted and live a happy and fulfilled life as an individual which is the opposite sex to the one assigned at birth.

The words transman or transwoman might be used, where a transman is a female who makes the transition to become a male and transwoman who is a male that makes the transition to become female. Their physical body is out of alignment with how they feel mentally and emotionally. Many transsexuals make the huge decision to undertake gender reassignment surgery. Those who have made the transition (who do not feel they come under the heading of transgender or transsexual) post surgery, may simply feel at ease and identify as a 'man' or 'woman'. Many may continue to come under the heading of 'transman' or 'transwoman' as they may not wish to ignore the journey they underwent in order to find their true selves. Therefore they will raise awareness of those who are suffering in the same way they did before making the transition.

JACK JIMENEZ'S STORY

"I have known I was a lesbian my entire life. I have a scar on my knee from jumping off a swing to impress the girl next door when I was five years old. I'm also a transman, but I still identify as a lesbian. I was raised as a woman, and very involved in the gay community, so I wouldn't know the first thing about being a straight man. Frankly, from what I have seen of straight men I wouldn't want to be one anyway.

Like many, I was bullied, not physically, but screamed at when I went to the Prop 8 rallies, which was expected. My uncle once accused me of trying to go after his wife and told me if I wanted to act like a man he would beat my ass like a man, this was before I was even transitioning. She had been my aunt since I was thirteen and it was completely bogus, but those sorts of things have come up. I feel almost guilty because I have been pretty lucky compared to a lot of other members of our community.

When I came out it was like I could finally breathe. Mom found a letter I'd written my girlfriend when I was fifteen so she already knew, but I didn't come out all the way until I was eighteen. I come from a really small town, and in High School I would have been out if not for all the rednecks and everyone knowing your business all the time. I kind of feel like I took the easy way, but what choice did I have? I was the only open lesbian in that town for years, and everyone knew about it and everyone talked about me when they found out. As soon as I graduated I came dancing out of that closet where I had hidden the real me for so many years because I knew I wouldn't have to be stuck with those people anymore.

I just decided that I was going to start living my life as me, and didn't give a damn what people thought about it. I was fortunate to realise at a young age that I don't have to be anything anyone expects me to be, I only have myself to answer to.

My coming out went much better than I thought it would. It didn't really matter what the reactions were, just being out and honest about myself was so freeing. I ended up working at a place with a lot of people I went to High School with. This was the first summer after graduation, and as soon as they found out they were like "Why didn't you tell us!?" I kind of wanted to be like "Well, because you're all catty bitches and would have treated me like shit at school anyway, and then smiled to my face after graduation like now..." but overall the response was pretty positive. I sealed the closet door well and truly shut and now I experience freedom. There's nothing more freeing than realising that you don't owe anyone anything and you don't have to be anything for anyone but yourself.

I now have a fantastic relationship with everyone except my uncles. My entire family has been really supportive, especially after I came out as transgendered also. My great-aunt couldn't come to my gay wedding in 2008 because she didn't believe in it; however she now proudly introduces me as her nephew. The only issue with family I have experienced is my two uncles. The one that accused me of trying to get with my aunt called me Frankenstein after finding out I was transman. In complete fairness to him, he is trying though, he took me out for a

220

beer shortly after that and has slowly started inviting me to do guy things with him. That is a big sign that he's working on it because he has very specific beliefs about the traditional roles of women and what they should and should not be allowed to do. He's not the type for apologies so that means a lot, and if that comes in the form of a beer then that's fine. My other uncle and my aunt have nothing to do with me. I have seen them twice in like five years, both times by accident. They did it right though, they never said anything bad to me, just cut me off. I'm completely happy with that.

I am at peace with myself and with God. My faith says God loves me. My culture can bite me. I won't live crammed in the closet anymore for anyone.

I love being a part of the gay community, and the majority of the people I have met in it. However, I get a lot of crap for being trans, people want to box me in as a straight man and I am not. I think people need to remember this is the GLBT community, and as such, our trans brothers and sisters are all a part of that. People in the gay community can be very judgemental. Being a transman is very controversial, especially among lesbians.

I have suffered some turmoil though, not over being a lesbian but by being trans, it is totally different. I find that I am too male for most lesbians, and whilst being pre-op I was too female for straight girls. I wondered daily if I was to spend the rest of my life alone because I chose to live as who I was inside. I did go on to meet a couple of Ms. Right's; but things didn't work out for one reason or another. I've been fortunate as I haven't had any problems with people over my relationships.

I was asked that given a choice if I could take a magic pill that would change me to be heterosexual, would I take it. My answer: HELL NO. Popeye said it best, "I am what I am and that's all that I am". Especially since I started transitioning, I'm finally living my life for myself and as I said before, I'll never live crammed inside that tiny little closet for someone else's comfort ever again".

The term 'crossdresser' has been defined as someone being born as one gender but identifying more with the opposite gender. They feel comfortable with the gender they have been assigned but prefer to wear the clothes of the opposite sex. The majority of crossdressers may in fact be heterosexual, they do not feel that they need or want to be like the opposite sex physically or mentally. The term crossdresser excludes people who wear the clothes of the opposite sex for any other reasons. This group does not include drag queens and female impersonators or anyone who crossdresses for a profession. Women can cross dress by adopting certain items that might be more in line with men and men can do the same thing. Although there might be a stereotype created for a cross dresser do not be fooled as I have heard of males who are in very masculine professions such as the building trade who cross dress as it is part of their identity.

DARYL FORD'S STORY

"I have to start by saying I am straight; there is no doubt about that. I am in my forties, have a masculine physique and I have a successful job in the construction industry. I have a beautiful home, a dream car, plenty of money thanks to my hard work and a wonderful wife and children. I have been married for fifteen years and I love my wife and children dearly. I know that we all have secrets, and mine is that I like to wear my wife's underwear.

I don't go in for the whole make up thing, and I don't try on her clothes or anything like that. I have always liked the feeling of the silky material against my skin and as I don't have a bad shape I don't think it looks all that bad on me either. I cannot put my finger on where this stems from only that I have felt like this a very long time. Before I met my wife, and when I was a lot younger I was in a relationship with a girl who was happy for me to wear her underwear and her stockings and suspenders during our love making however, she was the only one I did that with. When we broke up she called me a freak, I don't think she meant it, she just wanted to hurt me so I have kept it to myself since then. I have wanted to tell my wife on so many occasions in the hope it might spice things up in the bedroom department. We have always had a healthy and happy love life but I am always left wondering that if she found out then she might just throw in the towel. I dress up when she is out with the children or I am home early from work. I have become quite calculating about what underwear I wear so that she doesn't notice anything odd when she is doing the laundry.

I have read up on crossdressing using the internet so I can get a better idea of what has made me the way I am. Some men have said it is a type of play acting like when we are kids, girls want to be Cinderella and boys want to be Action Man or Spiderman. I suppose it might be the same for me in adulthood, I don't want to be a woman but for those few hours it is fun to pretend. It is a world apart from wearing my shirt, tie, jeans and reinforced boots with my hard hat and high vis jacket; it is different from what I normally wear.

I am glad to have found out that it is not unusual and I am not a freak of nature as there are other men who do this, straight men. I have nothing against being gay, I have gay friends that I was friends with in school who came out in university but I am straight. I am now comforted in knowing that I am not alone and hope that someday our wives might understand what we are going through".

TRANSVESTITE

A transvestite was always thought to be a person who wore the clothes of the opposite sex to gratify a sexual pleasure but as we have moved on it has become apparent that transvestites are crossdressers and this is the preferred term for those who are comfortable with their assigned gender but feel more comfortable wearing the clothes of the opposite sex. The correct term, for those who use the clothing of the opposite gender for fetish or sexual gratification is transvestic fetishism and not transvestism. I know it sounds complicated, stay with me.

PAUL HANCOCK'S STORY

"I am a bisexual male although I prefer to be with women, I find men attractive however my preference for a life partner would come in the

form of a woman. I would class myself as a transvestite and not a crossdresser, although personally, I'm not 100 per cent on how you define the difference. I don't just wear women's clothes but I also put on make-up and have false breasts.

I am not married and never have been and don't have any children. In the past I have told some partners and some have completely supported me and even bought me clothes. There have been others who didn't want me doing it around them; fortunately I have never had any bad reactions. Now I tell any possible partners about being a transvestite so they know from the start. If they can't accept what I do or who I am, it would never work long term. Honesty is definitely the best policy.

I have told those who are close to me about my bisexuality and my dressing in female clothes and the reaction has been positive and my friends and loved ones are there to support me. I have not told my parents however. Although there is such a thing as unconditional love, there are some things I guess you don't need to share with your parents. They wouldn't have a problem if I'm honest; it's me who has the problem. The longer I have known a person, the harder it is for me to tell them, the shorter the time then the easier it is.

I must have done a good job when I picked my friends as they have all accepted what I do and what I am. There have been only positive reactions and I know this is rare and I am very blessed. There have been a few surprised reactions and some have needed a while to come to terms with it but they have all stuck by me. I hid the real me for a long time before deciding to tell people, no matter what the consequences, but all it does is eat you up inside, but when I told my first friend about myself the weight just seemed to lift from my shoulders.

When I am in my female clothing my name is Kirsty. As a bisexual I have had experiences with men, most of these encounters have been while I have been dressed as a woman. Although they are gay, and I am Kirsty, I am still able to satisfy a gay man. My dressing up is not just for the bedroom though, normally when I dress up it is for a night out on the town. As Kirsty I feel more like myself and relaxed, so I would have to say it is a form of expressionism.

When I am Kirsty I visit the gay scene or pubs that are gay friendly. There is also a transwoman club that meet fortnightly I sometimes go there because I feel accepted and I will not get stared at. I found out about them through my local Gay Advice Centre.

A piece of advice to anyone who is exploring their new found feeling of transvestism is to get online and speak to others. I found just by speaking to other like minded individuals gave me the confidence to go for a night out on the town as Kirsty. I joined a website that had a section for guys who liked to dress as women, from the pictures I posted I received a lot of positive responses.

I would not dream of changing for anyone. If I had my time over again then I would not wish for anything different, I love what I do and who I am, it is part of what I am, and without it I would be incomplete, I would only be half a person".

DRAG QUEEN

The term drag is applied to men who dress wearing female clothing and make-up in a flamboyant and 'over the top' style in order to create striking caricatures of women. 'Drag queens' are an art form. They merely wish to entertain. They are seen as theatrical and funny and usually perform as stage artistes for a living; they can become local, national or international celebrities. Those who are involved in this profession do not necessarily have to be gay, they may be natural born entertainers who feel comfortable with themselves to adorn the wig and high heels and get a sense of job satisfaction through making people smile. Barry Humphries who plays the remarkable and internationally loved Dame Edna Everage is straight, he also plays other characters in order to entertain his audiences but it is Dame Edna who has been his ticket to a successful career. There are some who take exception to the term drag queen and prefer to be called female impersonators. I am not sure why this is exactly, perhaps it comes down to sexuality, drag queens might be men that are gay and female impersonators might be straight men who do pretty much the same job. It could be that a 'female impersonator' tones down the flamboyancy in order to make the character more believable and less of a caricature.

225

Another interesting concept thrown into the mix during my research came from a close friend who says that some female impersonators feel that they are too superior to be referred to as a 'mere drag queen' on the basis that they perform away from the gay scene and have become well known and very successful whereas a 'drag queen' might be just as talented or even more so. Nevertheless since they play the pub and club circuit they are seen as 'drag queens'.

Take for example Fanny Dazzle, born in a trunk at the London Palladium, not in her home city of Cardiff, South Wales. She is a true gender illusionist of our time and is pure showbiz through and through. She is the illegitimate love child of two prolific showbiz icons of the 1960's, so Fanny has the business we call show running through her veins. Having worked all over Europe, Fanny has now settled in Cardiff because she is Welsh first and London Palladium second. She entertains crowds each and every night in Cardiff and across the UK in her one woman show. Her comic timing is second to none, and majesty of grandeur in a voice that could stop traffic – literally. Versatility should be her middle name - but she hasn't got one.

Beneath the hair and make up of this fictitious character there is a very real person, a man called Alan who has made it his work to make people laugh, feel good and laugh at life.

FANNY DAZZLE'S STORY

"Thinking back to when I was coming to terms with my sexuality there were very few gay role models. I knew from watching television that there were men who were attracted to other men, so I never really thought I was the only one, but growing up in Cardiff, South Wales I knew I had to keep myself to myself. I remember I would wear my big coat over my school uniform so I could go into The Kings Cross which is one of Cardiff's oldest gay pubs.

Today, you might say I am part of the furniture of that old pub and the gay scene in general. When I created Fanny Dazzle it was through pure chance. Before we start, I will let you know that I am a drag queen, not a female impersonator. A female impersonator goes for the convincing
226

illusion of being a woman, they play the part as I do but with more finesse. Where as me, it's all done in some over exaggerated way, it's quite clear that I am a bloke in a frock! I started out as a comedian/singer as myself and then things changed.

I never thought I would be making my living as Fanny. I was being paid higher sums of money to be funny and sing the odd song as Fanny than being myself – bloody right too; hair and make up cost a fortune. I started off buying my clothes rather modestly in normal clothes shop, but needed a major overhaul if I was going professional. One day my friend whisked me off to London, he took me to a retailer that created made-to-measure dresses and gowns for drag queen and female impersonators. They cost a fortune. I couldn't buy one because at the time I just wasn't earning it. I was told that if I bought the dress it would make me enough money to cover the cost of the dress and a hell of a lot more besides. The decision was made and I bought it. They were both right, that dress was the best investment I had ever made. It was beautiful and when I wore that dress I elevated myself from a meagre drag queen to an artiste that could compete with the best of them.

*I now have a wardrobe of fabulous gowns, and I have an outfit for every occasion. When I am Fanny, I think of myself as a slightly crazy woman from the South Wales Valleys who has won the lottery and hasn't got a f****** clue what to do with it. I have always had a penchant for Hollywood glamour, and this is clear when you see Fanny.*

There have been many highlights in my career as Fanny Dazzle, the only purpose of her is to help people have fun, be accepted, get entertained and have a good time. One of the greatest experiences was when I was asked to perform on the main stage at Cardiff Mardi Gras around ten years ago. I entertained around 40,000 people – just my luck that it happened to be particularly busy that year. My entrance was fantastic as the entire crowd shouted "Hello Fanny!" my response came "You have just made this old queen very happy... 40,000 of you all shouting for fanny!!!" I played my part and then did what Fanny does best - I finished with a ballad. For those ten minutes or so I felt I was in my own little world, for that short time I was a star. The ballad I sang was

227

Perfect Day, and it was for me. I have sung that song a good few times since, but nothing beats the first time I sung it, which will always be very special to me.

It's not all glitz, glamour and sequins you know. There are lowlights too, and boy there have been many. The worst thing that can happen professionally is when you are in the middle of a performance with your friend and colleague (another drag queen whom you are part of a double act with), and as you sing "Let me entertain you" some bitter old queen from the audience shouts "Well f****** go then!". Well all that did happen, and it actually happened to me. I travel across the UK with my show and one night we performed an evening of cabaret in Coventry. Again nothing went right; my singing was not up to the usual standard and no-one laughed at my jokes. That was the longest forty minutes of my life. I came off stage and actually cried, and vowed never to perform again... but I did! You pick yourself up, dust yourself off and start all over again.

There is a special place in comedy for drag queens and the female impersonator. The purpose is to make people laugh and bring people together, some make fun and over exaggerate the female form and some worship and glorify it... and some just look like a bloke in a frock at a family party. It can take me anywhere from about forty minutes to two hours or more to get ready. If I only have an hour then it takes me an hour, if I have longer then I'll use it. Usually an hour does it.

There is a thrill for me when I adorn some outrageously glamorous and over the top gown, but that is more to do with the theatricality of it than the femininity aspect. In actual fact as quick as it goes on, it comes off again. When people meet me and I'm Alan they are quite surprised when they find out who I am... they expect me to be in the dress... when I'm in the supermarket... and it's 1:30 in the afternoon. It is just what I wear to work as a mechanic would wear overalls. The real thrill is in the entertaining. To those I don't know they might think I am a crossdresser, a transvestite or a man who desperately wants to be a woman. I am none of those things; the closest I get to crossdressing is when I wear a cardigan.

228

When you are a man wearing a dress you clearly have more freedom to be outrageous, it's what people expect. Being Fanny allows me to say the things I wouldn't dare say when I am myself. My favourite performances are non-gay events or bookings. I can be very flirty with the men and it amuses me hugely because they know I am a bloke but they accept it because of the dress and they know it is entertainment... it is all quite bizarre.

My advice for anyone looking to pursue a career as a drag queen or female impersonator is... just do it! Don't think about it too much; if you really want it then just go for it. You do need to practice your singing; rehearse your routine and you need to have your repertoire in order. The comedy will only come through practice and actually getting out there and doing it. Get an act and work on it. Yes, getting the look right is important, but I didn't start off where I am now. The looks will only carry you for about fifteen to twenty seconds, and if you haven't got an act then you are up Shit Creek without a paddle.

My family are completely supportive of my sexuality and my profession and they have all at some point watched me perform, one of my brothers had no choice because Fanny attended and performed at his birthday party. I have settled down with my partner, Trevor who also became my ball and chain in October 2009. He has three children which are obviously not my own, but I do look on them as mine. I have come to love them as if they are, they have all seen me perform on many occasions and are more than supportive, they actually understand - they know its just my job.

When I married Trevor I never in a million years contemplated wearing a dress. It was me marrying Trevor, not Fanny but Alan. Some people have asked why I didn't wear the white dress, if only for a laugh, but being a drag artiste is a job and how I earn my living. It only defines what I do to earn money and as for a laugh, I took my wedding very seriously as I did my wedding vows. Our wedding was so special; I wanted it to be fun but not a circus and most definitely not a laugh. It was the happiest day of my life so where is the humour in that".

You can find out more about Alan and his interpretation of the gay scene in Chapter Five.

Drag Kings & Faux Queens

The term 'drag kings' applies to females who take on the role of a male and faux queens is a term that applies to women who perform as drag queens. So to confuse you a little more, faux queens are women who are pretending to be men dressing as women. Now you really are confused. If you want better clarification watch the hugely funny movie, Connie and Carla starring Toni Collette and Nia Vardalos. This is one of my favourite movies of all time and you read more about this movie by visiting **www.ClosetsAreForClothes.co.uk**.

CHAPTER SIXTEEN

Conclusion — The Meaning Of Life

I mentioned 'The Meaning of Life' at the beginning of the book. It is one of those questions that everyone ponders at sometime or another. Monty Python even made a film about it.

What is The Meaning of Life? The simplest answer is - you. You are probably sat there now thinking "Uh, that's lame, or corny or cliché", it is what it is. We have all been put on this planet for a reason. There is not one person on this earth whether they have been ordained to a position of great importance or any type of wealth through birthright that is better than you. The contribution you make to life exists only because of you. When you do good things it makes you feel good, and if you stop and think it actually makes others feel good too, and in turn they may go on to do good things because of you. It's not rocket science, its human nature. It's about enjoying life and being kind.

Another good question that people ask: "Is there a cure for being gay?" The answer to that is no. There is no cure because it is not an illness. It will take more than Lemsip Max Strength to cure being gay. It is something you are born with; you haven't been cursed, jinxed or created inferior to anyone else. I have never met a person who has chosen their sexuality; I have met those who have recounted a same sex experience. The punishment and isolation we can experience for being gay leads me to question why anyone would say they are gay for the attention. Growing up I would have given anything to be straight, and there are others who felt the same. There comes a point where you feel comfortable with being in the skin you are in and then it doesn't matter. It is only when you have the security of knowing that your family and friends still love and respect you that you will experience this euphoria. You smile without reason, your outlook becomes brighter and you shut out the rest of the world who might have a problem because you have everything you need. You don't need to be like everyone else, you can have more than everyone else, being born the same would mean not having to hide the real you. When I was younger, and if I had my way I would have chosen to be straight, but now I realise, if I had my time over again I would be gay. I am happy now, and I would go through it all again. In actual fact if I had my way I would have been born a little bit taller, a tiny bit slimmer and with thicker hair, but you know what, I have got over it.

There are people out there that believe that homosexuality can be 'cured'. The simple suggestion or endeavour to change someone's sexuality will be mentally damaging to that person. It will diminish self-worth, self-esteem and fighting against the genetic make up will only lead to mental illness. There is nothing to fight as there is nothing wrong. Some faiths and groups are of the opinion that it can be cured; again you are as likely to make a gay person straight as you are to make a straight person gay. I understand what it is like to have religious beliefs and to understand that others of the same faith preach about changing so that we can be 'normal' and live without sin.

Sexuality cannot be changed. It's like asking someone to change their skin colour, their eye colour or hair colour. You can do it with make up, contact lenses and hair dye but underneath you will still have your true colours underneath. Our sexuality is deeply embedded within all of us, and I believe it extends further than simply dictating what gender we find sexually attractive.

A friend's father went on a course recently and during the break a conversation started about a recent newspaper story of a mother who had disowned her son because of his drugs addiction, stealing to fund his lifestyle. Some agreed that they would do the same; others took pity and assumed it was just a bad crowd, and a phase. As the conversation moved on to their own families, he was most surprised by the course trainer who responded "I think I would prefer my son to be gay than be a criminal". Having a gay son himself, he went on to tell them about this book being written to help those struggling with their sexuality, and educate those who have no idea of what it is like to be gay – such as those who believe it is better to have a gay child than be a criminal.

On another course, my friend's colleagues were laughing and ridiculing the head of a rival organisation (who was not present and is apparently gay but not very vocal about his sexuality). They supposed he was 'as camp as a row of pink tents', 'a slime ball', 'batting for the other side' and so on. My friend sat there quietly, ignoring their ignorant views of gay people. This went on and on until she became so incensed she said "Why don't you just call him gay, if you think he is gay, instead of the innuendos and snide remarks about his sexuality". She went on to say "I have a gay friend and he is one of the nicest people you would ever wish to meet. In fact, I think everyone should have a gay friend!" She has been of this opinion a little after my coming out, my caring nature and my quick wit, that has been remarked upon since I was a child, is partly to do with my sexuality and my respectable upbringing. I wouldn't change me in any way and neither would those who love me.

The only way that you will be totally happy and at peace is to love yourself. As you love yourself, others will not be able to help loving you too. You deserve only happiness and thankfully it is yours to take, all you have to do is reach out and grab it.

Just before the end of the book, I though you might like to read a few more stories from real individuals just like you who have dealt with issues and moved on happily.

Katie Lane's Story

"I realised that I was bi-sexual in June 2008; I knew the date because I was going into High School. It was then I finally came to terms with who I really was. I'd been thinking about it for a few months before, I had a strong attraction to my best friend. She had just come out as being bi-sexual, she always looked at me and said "there's no way you're straight". It was not that I chose to believe her; it was that I knew she was right. I have learned that the person's gender doesn't matter, as long as I love them that's okay with me.

I have been bullied for it but it cannot be considered to be outright bullying, I suppose. It's more the looks I get from people for wearing a t-

shirt supporting gay rights or rainbow related issues. If I give other girls hugs people tend to cringe or find it weird, I also get the old "its Adam and Eve not Adam and Steve" hollered at me, and that hurts when someone says it. It's as if they are saying that I was made incorrectly on the production line before I was given life. It is hard to hear.

I attend a school that is fine with being gay so it has never really been a problem. If someone were to have a problem with it then frankly I do not care. It's them that need to deal with it. I came out in school and nobody cared really, it's that attitude I respect.

When it came to my parents however it was a nightmare because I had double the trouble, I have four of them. My mom said when I told her, "it's easier in this world to be heterosexual" and I replied "well that's not going to change me". My stepdad was pretty cool about it; he sat and held me while I cried after my siblings had started bashing bi-sexual people because they "should just pick a gender". They didn't know about me but it still hurt a lot. My dad didn't really understand what it was so he had a bit of learning to do and my stepmom was totally dismissive and told me that I had the rest of my life to figure everything out. Yeah, like it's that simple.

I told my mom in the car ride home, she was driving and I told her that I had a girlfriend, so I went on to tell her about her. I felt like for some reason I had to have an actual girlfriend for her to understand that I wasn't confused or going through a period of self-discovery, or embarking on a phase that would result in my being heterosexual. She told me that if I was transgender or anything similar, I had to tell her now because she would have a really hard time accepting it if I was. When it came to telling my dad we were both up way past our bed time, this was a Saturday evening and we were doing what we always did on Saturday evenings, watching SNL. It was really nice and I enjoy spending quality time with my dad. I just wish my parents understood it a little better. I love them and they love me but they should have an idea of what I'm experiencing and the culture I belong to.

Coming out was like taking a big sigh of relief, sometimes I felt so vulnerable because I was finally being upfront and honest with them

234

about who I was and that leaves you feeling exposed and quite scared. My parents treat me as they always did but some times they push me away when I say something about gay people needing rights too. They almost remark that "they're fine". My dad is always happy to talk about it; he will always discuss gay politics when it is being featured in the media.

The way I now handle my bi-sexuality is as follows. I only remain friends with the people that support and understand me because it's a huge part of my identity; my stepsister however is not a very nice person if I'm honest. She knows that I'm bi-sexual and yet still feels the need to call things "gay" if they are uncool or bad and she refers to gay people as "fags" and various other derogatory terms. She knows how it upsets me therefore I have put up a barrier; this is the only way I can handle her sort. When it comes to religion I was devoutly Catholic until I was being repeatedly told by members of the church that God hated me and my kind. My own Priest said that "gay love is wrong", I haven't attended church since. If God does exist then surely he doesn't hate me.

I am happy being me and I continue with my studies and I am going to make the life that I deserve".

KAITLIN CRISLER'S STORY

"I think I have just now come to terms with everything, but I pretty much made out with my best friend Sasha in Junior School all the time. I haven't really been bullied by anyone as such but some people don't understand that it is something that they are privileged to know about me, it's not something to hang over my head as blackmail.

My coming out was slightly strange. I had been seeing my girlfriend behind my grandparents back for nine months when we were in a tragic car wreck where I broke my back. I was put on a morphine drip to numb the severe pain; I have since re-named morphine, truth serum. I told them everything while blissfully unaware. My family was actually really cool with it, they were more disappointed that I had lied and didn't think they would understand. Some make it a point when I'm around that they don't want to talk about my sexuality - that's families for you.

235

I am still at school and scared to come out of the closet, I always tried to be with guys because I was scared of the criticism I would receive but you can't fight what you know you are. I am glad that my close family know though, it's liberating and yet I felt exposed at the same time, kind of vulnerable. It did actually go better than I expected, but who can really be mad at someone in a hospital bed?

I have a great relationship with my parents, Mom is a lesbian so she understood and Dad is pretty cool about it. I have one friend who knows about my sexuality but denies it to herself because she hates gays and we have known one another since we were in diapers. Despite the good and the bad it is the best thing I have done, I don't have to constantly lie about who I am to people, especially those who are close to me.

I used to struggle with my faith, but if there is a God then I believe he made me this way. I didn't choose to love a woman instead of a man it was the way I was created therefore, I am what I am. There have been ups and downs along the way as I came to terms with myself. I became really depressed, unable to share my feelings with those who mattered, I felt like my life was essentially a lie. I had my life with my girlfriend where I felt fulfilled and my family life where I felt that I didn't fit in. I always tried to find guys attractive but couldn't, in fact it made me feel sick to my stomach and I felt like I knew I didn't want to be with a guy, it was all a part of trying to fit in.

I sometime socialise on the gay scene, however there is so much drama there, but at the same time there is a lot of unity. I've known many important and influential people in the gay community since I was four years old so I feel kind of at home when I'm around a lot of like minded people.

I am still young and have a lot of life to live, when I meet my Ms. Right and if we were to marry, there would definitely be a few people from my family who I would question inviting, but it's my happiness that counts not theirs".

"I knew I was gay for sure in eighth grade. I always had an attraction to men, but never knew what the word 'gay' meant. I decided to keep myself closeted for five years because I never knew how to deal with it. I was good at acting so it was easier at the time to act straight, than to embrace what I was feeling because I didn't think I was mature enough at the time.

I have never been bullied for being gay and have always been close to my friends, when I came out at the age of eighteen they just accepted me for who I was. I have experienced discrimination from one close family member and I remember another telling me she supported Proposition 8 through an email. Since then, our relationship has never been the same.

Coming out for me took five years which was from the time I was thirteen until I was eighteen. I had to assure myself that I wasn't confused and was really gay. I realised that I wasn't attracted to women and could appreciate a woman's body, but not in a sexual way. The truth was that I was and still am attracted to men. I came out after High School in the September of 2007. It was much easier in college because people are more accepting in most cases.

I came out to my mother three times and my father only once. My mom thought I was just confused, and to this day I still feel that she thinks that. We've had arguments over it, sometimes about how I walk, or even telling people I'm gay. She said I was trying to be something I wasn't and that this was just some kind of fad. She has hurt me emotionally on several occasions, and to this day, I pretend I'm fine with it, but my scars have not completely healed. I know and can feel that there is a certain level of shame with her. My father only had to be told once. He responded with "I'm not happy about it" and still doesn't acknowledge it to this day. I was only afraid to come out to my parents because I always knew I'd have support from my brother, other family members, and old and new friends. The parents were the hardest to tell and the last to find out. My mother's reaction was surprising because she always expressed that she was okay with the gays, but my dad was not surprising at all.

There was a certain sense of relief after coming out because I felt I wasn't lying to anyone anymore and I could live my life the way I'm supposed to. My relationship could be better with my parents, but I've expressed how I feel and a lot of the time they don't want to hear it. I still to this day have not brought any men home because I'm scared of what the family will think. I shouldn't feel that way, but I do. My strongest relationships are with my very close cousins, aunts and new friends I've made along the way. I can honestly say it is the smartest thing I have done because I was miserable trying to play a straight guy.

The first relationship I had was with a guy named Will. I was nineteen, he was twenty-two. He wasn't a good guy though. He was kind of a player and I had no time for that. He was bisexual, which there's no problem with, but he tried dating both genders at the same time and I couldn't have that. I do have ethics and morals, and that didn't fit with mine.

As far as religion goes, I do believe in God, but I don't believe in organised religion. I feel that religion just sends mixed messages with saying that we are all loved but only if you do certain things or abide by everything the Bible states. I know in my heart that God doesn't hate anyone because of their sexuality but for the kind person they are.

The only mental health issues I have experienced was with my weight. I ate my feelings and that's how I dealt with my closeted self. After coming out, I lost the weight and was really happy with myself. I have cut myself because I felt emotional pain from the things my mother said to me, but I'm over that now. Self harm is not something I would recommend.

I found solace when I visited the gay scene, being surrounded by those who understood me. It is like a safe haven from any discrimination against sexual orientation. I have straight friends who visit it too and they are completely fine with it. In fact, they endorse it.

I'm single right now. Not exactly looking but I know Mr. Right is out there. A lot of the gay guys who live near me are usually attracted to the bright lights of the bigger cities such as New York, Los Angeles or San Francisco, and I can understand why, our culture is widely accepted there and I plan to leave and venture there and start a life of my own. I feel sad that I have to do that but I know that I can embrace the real me in a bigger city".

KRISTIE MYNATT'S STORY

"I knew that I was lesbian since being in kindergarten. I know that seems a little early and of course I didn't really know what it was, I just remember looking at the other kids and knowing that I was different to rest.

I was never bullied for being gay, I guess I was too intimidating to people who might have wanted to bully me so I was lucky on that score. I dated some guys in High School but I always knew I was gay, I thought that's how I was supposed to live - as a straight person. I knew that I was gay, I have always known so I decided to bite the bullet and just be myself.

I came out only after I had outed my brother, Kevin to our mom. I thought it was about time she knew about us both being gay so I just casually said, "Mom, Kevin is gay (long pause) and so am I". She was fine about it; he was away at the time so he had that to come home to. I never really had to tell anyone else as I guess they just assumed I was gay – and I have never denied it.

It was the best thing I had ever done, and it was like a weight had been lifted from my shoulders. The whole experience of coming out went better than I thought, Mom was fine with it and Dad disowned us for a while, but just needed a bit of time to get used to the idea of not just having one gay child, but two.

My mom is great, she is the support we both need and we love her dearly. It took Dad a while to get used to it but after the birth of my daughter he has come to except it. Our family just accepted it. It didn't matter to me if they did or didn't. I wouldn't consider myself a trusting person; I keep people at arms length so I don't have to keep getting hurt.

When it comes to religion I have it sorted. I have a close relationship with God. I know in my heart God makes no mistakes and I'm not a mistake and neither are the countless other gay, lesbian, bisexual or transgender people. I put God first in my life always. Without him I am nothing anyway. My religion is Christian and I attend a Methodist Church so everyone is pretty open to it and if their not they don't say anything. Our Preacher tells of God's love for everyone and everything – it's not exclusive to certain people. I am proud of who I am, but if I had a choice in life I would have never chose to be gay – I don't think anyone would.

When it comes to being gay I have created a few of my own theories. I think you are either gay or you're not. I don't really believe you can be bisexual; it's more to do with curiosity. It's like being straight, you are or your not and there is no in-between. There are some young kids who think it is cool to say they are gay or bisexual. I have witnessed this myself – they might experiment to see what it is like, but why bother. I know I sound hypocritical here but I grew up thinking I had to be straight and therefore tried to condition myself to living the straight life until I realised that there is a place for me in the world. I have noticed that a lot of people come out as being gay when they have suffered sexual assault. I was sexually assaulted at the age of seven but I remember knowing I was gay even before then; I just had an attraction to girls.

I met the love of my life ten years ago. We have a two year old daughter together and would love another child to complete our little family. My partner, Cassaundra and my little girl are my life. I knew from the very beginning that she was the one for me. It took over six months to get her to go out with me, but with patience she could soon see that I was right for her. She is five years younger than me so it was not exactly easy for us to go out together with people looking at us. I waited for her though and would have waited longer. I could spend all day talking about her, she is everything to me. We would love to cement our union to one another and have a legal marriage but we
240

never see that happening, but that will not stop us from having a ceremony. What the straight people don't seem to understand is I don't need a piece of paper to tell me I love someone".

~~The End~~

The Beginning

CHAPTER SEVENTEEN

Coming Out The Other Side — My Story

Lifting A Huge Weight

As a Life Coach the first exercise I ask my clients to carry out is to write their life story, nothing too big, just a bit of background that will fill half to a whole page of A4. This will usually bring any highlights and lowlights in their life to the foreground and will emphasise any significant events. As this exercise involves a lot of soul searching I think it only fair that I do the same. I have decided to write about my highlights, lowlights and significant events in order for you to get an idea of me. As a client you would not be asked to write as much as I am about to share with you, nevertheless, it is only fair that you know all there is to know about me should you decide to choose me as your Life Coach. One of the first things my mother said when I told her I was becoming a Life Coach was "You are too young to be a Life Coach". She is very supportive and always has been, but, like so many parents she worries that things will not work out or sees the dangers rather than the positives. I have lived, loved and lost, feeling the pain of bereavement, and pain at the hands of others, so yes I can say I have lived. Despite the bad things that have happened I still get up everyday with a smile on my face, while counting my blessings for being alive, healthy and having such wonderful people in my life.

Starting At The Beginning

We never think of ourselves as being special do we? We go through life encountering such brilliant opportunities, and experience the gut wrenching heartache of those dismal events that are simply a part of life. Those events are the ones that if they don't kill us, they should

243

theoretically make us stronger. Well, I am glad to say that I am special. Firstly, when I came into the world in the winter of 1982 I received the biggest lottery prize in the world. My prize did not come in the way of money, in its place I was blessed with the two greatest parents that ever walked this fair planet. For many people I know, life's biggest lottery is the parents that we have been blessed with.

I was born at home, in fact in the same house my mother and her brother had been born so to me that's pretty special. By the time I was seven I had planned my funeral, that is pretty darn special too if not a bit creepy. I was born gay – special, I have a large loving family – special, I have lived in three countries – special (and lucky) and I met the man of my dreams first time around – special (and scary). So yeah, I am special. All of us are special in our own unique way. I have always respected those who speak their minds; because it takes great skill to get your point over without being rude. I believe myself to be straight forward yet complex, I am decent and respectable however I can be the crudest person in the room; I love chick peas but cannot stand humus, I am monogamous yet firmly believe you can read what's on the menu but you don't have to order. I am gay and although I believe life is too short - I would never consider a relationship with a woman. See, I'm in complete opposition to myself. In fact my favourite aftershave is Contradiction by Calvin Klein.

The first major and significant event in my life took place in 1983 when I was around thirteen months old and it was then I very nearly sealed my own fate. I was left playing in the living room while Nanny Beatrice who was Mam's mother, was in the kitchen boiling an egg. I somehow dislodged the safety gate that acted as a barrier between the lounge and the kitchen. Nanny hadn't seen me and before anyone knew I reached up and pulled the saucepan of boiling hot water down from the cooker right over me. I cannot remember much about it, but Mam tells me that she bundled me into the sink and doused me with cold water, I do vaguely remember fighting Mam off as she tried desperately to immerse me in cold water, but I do not remember the pain or anything else. I was immediately rushed to the Burns Unit of a hospital in Chepstow which was some distance away from my home. I was in the Intensive Care Unit for seven days, the doctors and my parents thought

244

that my time was up. Well as you can see I did pull through, the nightmare had only just started for my Mam, she grieved for two after that, she cried most nights at the thought that she nearly lost me. The shock was all too much, she mourned as if I had died and each and everyday Dad reassured her that I was alive and well and that I was alright. Although I was completely covered by hot water the only scars that remain visible are at the top of my left arm, with a little scaring to my right arm. I was very lucky, not just to pull through but not being heavily disfigured which would have been the result if my mother had not reacted and doused me in the cold water. It was she that saved my life that day. She brought me in to the world and she fought to keep me in it. It is a good job too or I would not be here writing all of this now. It was this turn of events that meant I was a bit of a 'clingy' child. Wherever Mam and Dad were, I was not far behind.

If It Doesn't Kill You Then It Makes You Stronger

I started school at the age of three; I took an instant dislike to the place. I would kick and scream every morning not to go to that awful place. It was a horrid school that was mainly full of horrid kids and it smelt funny. Schools do, don't they? Some of kids were alright, but it was the bad ones (and unfortunately there was quite a lot of them) who ruined it for me. Mam broke her heart having to leave me there because she knew I hated the place, but I had to go. She did everything she could to help me settle; allowing me home for lunch to break up my day at school, but this resulted in me not wanting to go back.

As time went on, I did become more settled in school; although I was bullied and excluded by most of the other kids as far back as I have memory. I suppose that the kids could see things in me that I couldn't. I was treated differently from them, the girls were awful because I wasn't the typical candidate to represent the male of the species and the boys obviously saw this too - I couldn't fit in to either group. It was from an early age I learned how it felt to be ignored, whispered about just loud enough so I could hear, and be subjected to hurtful names that you would believe too unimaginable for kids.

I believed I was always destined to become an actor, it was the only thing I ever wanted to be and it was the only thing I was good at. I had been introduced very early on to the *Carry On* films. My best friends were Barbara Windsor, Sid James, Joan Sims and Kenneth Williams. Before I had reached my teens Dad introduced me to *Confessions of a Window Cleaner* and all the other *Confessions* titles (although a bit raunchier than the *Carry On* films - they were comedy gold). It was this early introduction to British Comedy that enabled me to be funny. I could make people laugh, especially the teachers. I was always selected to represent the school in the Welsh festivals (Eisteddfod in Welsh), acting, individual narration, and group choirs – anything requiring a performance. I had a knack for learning lines, I could easily memorise my lines and I had a good singing voice. I was a happy child even through the torment of others, and I still smiled each and everyday. It was my defence mechanism. I didn't want to stop smiling just because the others were so miserable.

My home life was brilliant, Dad worked in a foundry making aluminium wheels for cars, and he came home each evening reeking of industry, the smell of the oil and the distinctive odour that clung to the fabric of his clothes that came from the smouldering furnaces. He would rush in to have his bath and then lie on the living room floor with me and have drawing competitions and play "guessing games", he would draw an object and I had to guess it before he finished. It was this quality time that nurtured my talent for drawing and art.

The bullying went on in Primary School through to Junior School and it got a damn sight worse in the Comprehensive School. I had one saving grace during my time in Primary School, this came in the way of my Nanny Beatrice. She lived with us and Nanny did everything to keep me home; staying at home with her was a lot of fun. I was her companion and she doted on me, I was "Nan's Boy".

In December 1990, when I was seven years old I returned home from school alone. My brother was away on a field trip; my Mam and Dad were in work and not due home until 5:30pm. I was normally collected from school by Mam, as she only worked part time, or my brother, this time I was collected by my classmate's mother as they had to pass our house to get home.

I reached home, Nan wasn't at the door to greet me as usual, so I looked downstairs and she was nowhere to be seen. I went upstairs; her bedroom door was right at the top of the stairs, I could see she was lying on her bed groaning in pain. She kept telling me that she did not feel very well, I did not know what to do, I raced downstairs and grabbed for the phone, I called our local surgery to speak to our family doctor. I was told by the Receptionist that surgery was in session and she would get our doctor to give me a telephone call after surgery. By this point, I still didn't know what to do, I raced back up stairs and Nan was still groaning. I went to the window that looked out onto our street. I had to do something, Auntie Janice lived around the corner and I could just see her house in the next street from where I was standing but I kept thinking "it's just too far". I didn't want to have to lock the door and leave Nanny so I raced across the road to a neighbour, Christine. Christine came across, and stayed with Nan, she sat with her, stroking her hand, and just being a comfort to us both. Mam came home from work just as soon as she could and Nan was taken away by the ambulance and admitted to hospital for tests. The doctor kept asking Nan where it hurt and she just kept replying "all over". They made her comfortable for the night and said they would run tests in the morning. Auntie Joyce and Uncle Doug stayed with her that evening.

We were awoken in the early hours the following morning by the ringing of the telephone; the chimes from our Bakelite phone echoed up the stairs until I awoke. It was the hospital; they called to say my Nanny Beatrice passed away in her sleep. She died at the age of seventy-six years old, from an aneurism.

Auntie Joyce took charge of the funeral; she also stepped in where Nan had left off with me. She became more of a grandmother to me than an Auntie and more of a mother to Mam than a sister. Losing Nan at a young age made me question life and death, and my own mortality and that of my parents. At the age of seven my parents and I had come to the agreement that if I died before the age of eighteen I would be

247

cremated and kept at home in an urn and then buried when Mam or Dad passed away. We agreed that if I died after reaching eighteen years old then I would be put in with Nan and Grampy. I know this is a really weird thing to be arranging at the age of seven, but it gets better. In the event of Mam and Dad dying prematurely leaving me behind we arranged that I could go and live with Auntie Janice around the corner. Mam said I would be better off living with Auntie Joyce because she would spoil me more. So, it was agreed.

Although quite strange, this was a very real time for me even at such as young age. I had experienced bereavement way too early in life. I lived in constant fear until the age of sixteen that my parents would die and leave me in the same way my Nan had left. To top it all off I had the most dire school life, I was battling my sexuality and each day was more miserable than the last. Except for summer holidays and half terms, these were spent with my parents who were my best friends. The only people who didn't judge me or "exclude me from the group". I know you might be thinking I was a right miserable child but I wasn't. I was the complete opposite. I was always happy – singing, laughing and joking. To the outside world I was a bubbly, happy go-lucky child and today I am the same. I was only miserable at school and even then I tried not to let it show. I have always maintained a positive mental attitude and a good sense of humour, adopted through my time with my parents, I should think. You really needed to have a sense of humour to live in our house.

When I reached Comprehensive School all dreams of wanting to become an actor had well and truly been ripped away from me. I didn't know what I wanted to be or what I wanted to do. By this time my self-confidence and self-worth was running low, I just took each day as it came.

In March 1996 I went to my Welsh lesson after lunch and sat in my usual seat. We sat in class waiting for our teacher to arrive to find that he was unwell and we had a substitute teacher, a bright spark who thought it might be better to move the groups around as opposed to those set by our teacher. She grabbed the register and called out our names randomly, and as she did this, she allocated us new seats. I need to make it quite clear that I had a bad feeling about this from the start. So much so when she tried moving me I remained silent and tried to stay under the radar. But she was smart; she found me out and insisted I move to where she thought I should sit. I moved to my new seat as instructed; I was sat on a table of four. To my right there was a pupil that was also in my Art class, and having had Art that morning he had borrowed an art knife from our teacher so that he could complete some of his work at home. To my left there was a girl I had attended school with since we were both three years old. In a fit of boredom she began ransacking this boy's pencil case and found the art knife. Before I knew it she lashed out and stabbed me three times, once in the upper arm, once in the lower arm and once in the leg. I was fine for a while, then I started feeling hot and found myself sweating, I noticed my lower arm was bleeding so I asked to go to the toilet; I cleaned myself up and went back to class. Whilst I sat there I had a rush of pins and needles from the base of my spine all the way up to the top of my head. I touched the top of my left arm with my right hand, and I remember thinking that it didn't feel right. I pulled the neck of my school jumper so I could peer down and as I did I saw my blood drenched shirt sleeve. In a blind panic I ran for the door and rushed to the toilet. I cupped cold water in my right hand as I frantically tried to stop the blood; the feel of slippery sticky blood was more prominent than the water. Again, I panicked and remembered she had gone for my thigh, I quickly undid my belt and pushed my trousers to my knees, and thankfully there was no blood. Again returning to my arm I notice that there was more and more blood, as I tried to stem the flow of blood with cold water, the worse it became. I grabbed a tissue and tried to stay calm. When the bleeding had subsided I headed back to my class which was a small port-a-cabin. I opened the door which led into a dark corridor that joined the classroom. She just stood there in the corridor, I couldn't mistake those slanted eyes. I went into class and took my seat and was told by the fourth person on the table that she had been slung out for laughing and not for what she had done to me. When the teacher could see what had happened to my arm she sent me to the teacher next door. This was not much comfort, to me, she was a spinster and supposedly a Christian, but you wouldn't think so, she had a reputation for being insensitive at the best of times. By the time I reached her class I was in shock, I kept saying (in Welsh) "I didn't do anything! I didn't do anything!" She just snarled at me, "We'll see about that when we find out the facts of what happened!" She packed me off to the school Nurse who dressed my arm and then I was free to walk home. When I arrived home, Mam was at the door waiting for me, as I had called her from my mobile phone to say that I was on my way home. Needless to say Mam was not amused. In fact she was running with the wolves.

That night, and a few nights that followed apparently I shouted a lot in my sleep. I wasn't aware of this until Mam said. After the incident I didn't want to go back to that school because of what had happened and also because of the teacher's reassuring words, I thought I was in a whole heap of trouble.

The ironic thing is that I was right to feel uneasy about moving seats. My gut instinct told me something and I listened, unfortunately the power to listen to my inner voice was overruled by someone who apparently knew better.

The girl in question was later suspended, she didn't face permanent expulsion in the same way another pupil did a few months previously, when he stole a knife from the school canteen and scratched a teacher's car. This immediately taught me that it is not okay to destroy the personal possessions belonging to teachers; however as pupils we could cause real physical harm to one another and get extra time off school. I am glad that a Toyota Corolla or whatever it was had been held in higher esteem than me.

I went through the remaining years of school counting down each and every day until I could leave, this happened for two solid years. I had no intention of staying on to further my education, I just wanted out. I had no clue as to what I was going to do with the rest of my life.

Another significant event came when I ate the school curry one Friday afternoon. It was not something I would normally eat but I did all the same, which gave me a relentless bout of food poisoning. This resulted in no food for over a week and constant vomiting and diarrhoea. On my return to school everyone wondered where the little plump boy had gone, they thought he had left. I was a new person, the weight I lost – the 'puppy fat' my mother called it had gone for good.

Looking back over my time in school, I realise that although the popular 'chocolate' boys (named because they were what everyone perceived to be perfection, clear skin, popular, sporty – but in reality they were anything but; acne, bad mannered and only energetic when it suited them) managed to be off losing their virginity with the other 'easy' girls in my year with little regard for their own self-worth. Hearing the rumours of the schoolyard reinforced that although homosexual, and an outcast, my morals and self respect were in tact and that my self control was something that was to become my biggest asset, and strength. It was these 'chocolate' boys who were 'off being men and doing manly things' that would pass me in the school yard and casually shout "gay", "poof", "bender" and anything they felt necessary to boost their ego.

Sixth Form

Sixth form was a part of my life that very nearly didn't happen. Having had such a terrible time in school, I just wanted to leave, and to be as far away from the place as possible. However, not knowing what I wanted to do with my life I felt I had very few options. I remember completing the application form at home whilst looking back at the times I was taken to Primary School against my will with the exception of those few cherished days when Nan was able to save me from its clutches. I was transported back to Comprehensive School and heard all the name calling and feeling the emptiness at the pit of my stomach as I re-lived those moments. I looked back on the moment that my Welsh lesson left me blood soaked. Perhaps the idiots who made my life hell might have had better things to do than stay on in school. I came to the conclusion that I should submit my application and return to the sixth form. There was a voice inside that questioned if I was doing the right thing. I tried to be defiant; however I was left wondering "what if?" I didn't think that they would accept me back, but as sure as the little voice had said, I received a letter from the Head of Sixth Form inviting me back. I returned back to school in as much fear as I did on my first day when I was eleven. I had been right after all, the morons did in fact leave or were rejected and many of those who remained were good people.

The whole thing was quite bizarre. As a member of the sixth form we no longer sat on the floor for assembly - we had chairs, the finest plastic that government money could buy. We were in sixth form now and I was like a Queen. The freedom from structure and the lack of arseholes that sixth form offered allowed me to grow, and I went through an accelerated learning process in the subject of *Me*. I always knew who I was from a young age but it was here that I really had a chance to be me and the majority of those who returned to sixth form liked me. Keeping my guard well and truly up, I was cautious until I realised that there were no ulterior motives, no-one befriended me just so they could walk away and make fun of me behind my back, it was just... normal. It was normal, and I loved it. Many of those who returned to school were those who had at least made an effort with me in my last two years of GCSEs, and the others whom I did not know were of the same temperament. Finally, I was happy at school. I realised that I was liked by the majority of people, even from the time I first went into comprehensive school. The people that disliked me were the minority but I built them up to be the majority which caused me to withdraw from interacting with those who didn't have a problem with me.

At home I desperately wanted to tell someone about how I had been feeling as far back as I could remember. I was so close to telling them but I bottled out every time. My sister-in-law would stay over and some mornings we would be the only ones up. I would watch her while she did her hair and make up, I was fascinated by the whole process. We would drink tea and talk; she was like a sister to me, the sister I never had. I so very much wanted to tell her that I was gay, but I couldn't. I knew she would understand but I couldn't say the words in fear of choking on them, turning blue and being stuck in an urn.

Something I have failed to mention thus far is when I fell hopelessly head over heals for a guy in the year below. It happened way before sixth form, even before the stabbing incident. I was in fact fourteen years old and it was during the first week at school after the summer holidays, it was during the first year of my GCSE's. I was waiting at the school gate for my friend to arrive by bus when the guy in question strolled past with two of his friends. It was at that point that everything around me came to a standstill just like it does in the movies. From nowhere Karen Carpenter began singing 'Close to you' and I wondered to myself what the hell was happening. I'd never noticed him before but it didn't matter, I was in love! Well evidently it wasn't love, I was too young, and I didn't know what that type of love was. For the next two years I would see this guy walking around school, rushing back and forth to lessons and queuing at lunch. This was the strangest experience of my life because he was at every turn. I wished and prayed for the feelings to go away; I had managed for fourteen years without them so I was happy to continue. I did not want to feel the emotions I was experiencing; I didn't even know his name! Time went on, and the feelings and the emotions that came with them became natural, and emotionally draining to say the least. Even so, they never subsided, but I wished often that they would disappear.

To cut a long story short, as I moved into sixth form and made new friends, mutual friends then made it possible for us to talk and to become friends. It was all I wanted, yes I still had the same feelings for him that I had for two years, in fact they were even stronger, yet it was enough for me just to be friends. I did not want anything from him; in fact he had nothing he could give me except the friendship we built.

I then became part of a social world that I had no idea existed; there was plenty of partying and weekly visits to various pubs. Every Friday without fail we would all congregate in a small pub that was soon to be our second home. It was an old man's pub; the alcohol was so cheap they were practically giving it away. We kept the jukebox well stocked with pound coins and we had a tremendous time. Our Friday night gang would watch the seasons change from that old pub, with the jukebox securely behind us we sang, laughed and drank through the winter, while the weather changed we were unchanged, well so I thought.

As time went on there became a distance between us, and that came down to my sexuality. I knew I was gay, and perhaps although I never discussed it, it might have been obvious to others. My so-called "friends" eventually poisoned the mind of the boy I had become great

253

friends with. He was straight and I was gay, there was nothing more than that. The more they played on the fact I was gay the more he wanted to do a runner. I can't blame him; I might have done the same if I were in his position. We parted company, it was never done in any kind of way, he just removed himself from our friendship and that was the end of another chapter in my life. I was upset about it; I grew a thicker skin (no good moisturiser jokes please) and moved on. I had been through worse than that in my life so I was not going to let that hold me back.

It did make me wonder though. With some of the "friends" I had, did I need any enemies?

A New Beginning

With a positive mental attitude I sailed through sixth form. Yes, I experienced heartache at the hands of those I should have known better not to trust; nevertheless all in all I enjoyed it. I would re-live it all again. After waving goodbye to the best two years of my school life I was just as quickly waving hello to my adventures in Canada. Dad's work took us to live in Barrie, Ontario. A place filled with some of the nicest people on the planet. I soon learned that Canada was home to wonderfully warm, friendly people who opened up their lives and their homes to make us feel welcome in their part of the world. I felt safer in Canada than I had ever felt back home in the UK, the people were friendlier and the place was totally unthreatening. I occasionally walked around the streets of downtown Barrie at 11:00pm when I was a little home sick or couldn't sleep. The people would look me straight in the eye and greet me, as I passed.

The conditions of my visa meant I couldn't take part in any paid work which was all well and good because I was happy just to shop everyday. These plans were then scuppered when Dad's colleague secured me a position in the role of Production Assistant for The New VR, a local television station. I had six wonderful months there; the people were just the greatest and ever so slightly crazy. I soon became known as 'Richard from Wales' and was very popular with them. I fitted in immediately as I spent my days learning all there was to know about the ins and outs of running and working in a television studio. I loved watching the news being recorded and aired live, it just seemed more relaxed than the news I was used to, it was the longest time I had ever stayed quiet. As I looked on I often thought that it could have been me doing that had I just grown some balls and stood up to a few people.

It was February 2001 and Dad's work came to an end when the decision was made to close the Aluminium plant in Barrie. It was a shock for all concerned, especially the three of us as we had visions of a longer life in Barrie.

This episode was only a part of my new beginning, six short months. But the chain of events that were to follow my return from Canada was all part of the start of my new life.

Something else I have failed to mention before now is that I always thought from the age of eight that I was destined to be alone when I grew up. I was around the age of seven or eight when I knew that I was different from all the other little boys and girls, I knew I wasn't attracted to girls. Being aware of my feelings meant that I was almost sure that I was going to be alone in life. It was possibly due to the fact that I had lost Nanny Beatrice and therefore had an abandonment issue. It may have boiled down to the fact that the bullies had wielded a power that left me feeling worthless and insignificant. I perhaps thought it might not be possible to find love with the same sex. Was I really the only gay in this little Welsh village!? I conclude that there was a mixture of events that helped me believe I would live a solitary existence. Nan's passing, severely left its mark on me. The bullies made me feel unworthy to even breathe the very air they did and I didn't think it was possible to find love with another man. I had nothing against women, my mother is one, but I certainly didn't want to be with a woman, I thought I was destined for the single life. On the other hand, my parents were terrific role models for me on the relationship front. If I were to have a relationship then I wanted one like theirs. Mam had met Dad when she was fourteen years old. She took one look at him and not even knowing his name she decided that she was going to marry him. As I grew up and went through puberty I thought that if I did meet anyone then I wanted it to be like that for me. I wanted to meet the man of my dreams straight off. My parents met in a jukebox room while John Lennon serenaded them with 'Hey Jude'. If, and I say *if*, I was going to find someone then that is how I wanted it to be.

And it was.

Gordon Bennett Meets Mr. Arsey

Through sixth form I had spent a lot of time with Sarah, we were best friends at that time. I went to her home one day after she delivered the terrible news that her Nan, Mary, had terminal cancer. I had always been fond of Mary, I called her Mrs. Griffiths. I had a lot of respect for her as she was always very nice when I visited - it was after all her house and she was always very welcoming towards my coming and going. Sarah and her parents lived at home with Mrs. Griffiths in the same way we had with Nanny Beatrice. Mrs. Griffiths' home was a large manor house, and I had never been in a 'normal' house like it. I say normal because all my friends lived in semis, or very modest detached houses but this thing took the biscuit. It was beautiful; it sat right beneath Castle Coch, the Welsh fairy-tale castle built by the Marquess of Bute. It was grand; Mrs. Griffiths and her husband had bought it when they decided to set up home. I could not even begin to think how many times I could have fitted my house into it. I went to the house one night to see Sarah, it was then the rest of my life would change forever. It was like something out of Jane Austen. Sarah's mother asked if I wanted to say hello to Mrs. Griffiths who was upstairs resting. Sarah's mother went first and I followed, I took to the huge sweeping staircase and as I ventured forth I noted a dark figure coming down as we proceeded up. Sarah's mother stopped to speak to the man whose identity was not known to me and with that I stopped as they engaged in conversation. Someway through the conversation Sarah's mother introduced me to her Nephew, I did not know what to say and the only thing that came to mind was "Alright?" and he said it... that's right... nothing! Not a word. I said "Alright" and he said nothing. Granted, he did look at me when I addressed him; then carried on his conversation. My first opinion of him was something I cannot write for reasons of impropriety. After they had finished speaking he carried on down the stairs and we continued up, and that is when it happened. I turned back as we carried on up the stairs and I watched him go down and I said to myself "I am going to spend the rest of my life with him'". That was the day Gordon Bennett met Mr. Arsey. I had fallen in love. I didn't mean to and I certainly didn't want to, but there it was. His name was Andrew and that was my life partner, whether he liked it or not.

Andrew helped his parents in their business which was situated very close to Sarah's parent's business; I helped them out during Mrs. Griffiths' illness. You see Sarah's father and Andrew's father were brothers and Mrs. Griffiths their mother. Andrew visited his grandmother most evenings at her home. During her illness Andrew spent everyday with his grandmother. He adored her the same way I did my Nan. Mrs. Griffiths doted on him, I could see that. A few weeks passed, he bought me a Chocolate Fudge Sundae from Marks and Spencer's for my Birthday and the rest is history. We were friends for a while, all of three weeks I think and then we took it from there.

May 2001 came and went taking Mrs. Griffiths along the way, Andrew was devastated. In September 2001 I secured myself a position as a Customer Services Representative in a call centre, everything was moving in the right direction.

Another... New Beginning!

As if I hadn't experienced enough change, the plot went on to thicken as we heard news in November 2001 that the visas and paperwork came through for Dad's new job in South Africa. Andrew and I had been together for seven months by this time, but I had to pack up my life and move to sunny, yet windy Port Elizabeth in the New Year. I had very little choice in actual fact; my new job was a lot of fun and I worked with some wonderfully crazy, off the wall people, but it didn't pay enough for me to live alone so I had to leave. I was encouraged by my friends and other managers at work to leave right away so that I could enjoy Christmas. I gave my notice in work, only having been there two months but I decided to work all the way up until I was due to leave.

Grampy Tom, Mam's father, although I didn't know him he often told my mother that "you catch more bees with honey than you do vinegar". This served me well in my choice to leave my employer as it was this attitude that became a saving grace for me. Adopting Grampy Tom's instruction I was of the opinion that as the company had spent money training me then they should at least get their monies worth. This favour repaid itself in time.

After a heart wrenching goodbye, I said goodbye to my friends and family and the man that I had unexpectedly found. It was even more difficult as everyone saw us as just good friends, no questions asked. Had people understood how we felt then, perhaps we might have had more options not to part. The right time to *come out* had not shown itself; therefore I stayed silent and went with the flow.

South Africa was a million miles from the life I had known back home in South Wales. It was great that the Harris family were back on the road again. We had a beautiful apartment in Summer Seas, which was situated on the beach beside the Indian Ocean; a lovely car and I had a sun tan - for the first time in my life. I had all of this but still I was desperately unhappy. Andrew and I phoned one another everyday for three months, we wrote and sent cards back and forth. I knew this couldn't go on. I had to make a decision and choose between Mam and Dad or Andrew. I didn't want to leave my mother alone in a foreign country while Dad was at work all day, yet I needed to do what was right for me... or should that be right for us. You see, it is all well and good when you are on your own, you can please yourself but as soon as you meet 'the one' then it becomes *us*. One evening we plotted my escape from South Africa. The very next day I called Steve who was my immediate manager in the call centre where I had worked. It was thanks to him that I could return as he secured my old position back at my old desk. Andrew said he would move in with me to share the running costs at home, all I needed to do was break the news. I explained to Mam and Dad that I missed my home and my job and needed to live my life back home. I explained that Andrew being my best friend would move in to help out financially. I caught the next flight home and I knew that I had made the right decision.

A Change Of Scenery

After returning home, I called Tim; we had been friends in school and met just before our GCSE years. He told me that since I had been away he was visiting the gay scene in Cardiff. He said that he wasn't gay however he enjoyed the scene and we should go together. This was a 'shock horror' moment for me. I said very little during that phone call. It was like everything was coming at once.

Saturday night came and I descended head first into Cardiff's gay scene. It was a bit of a shocker, having kept my feelings deep inside myself for so many years I suddenly found myself emerged in a crowd of people who felt the same as me. A series of thoughts rushed through my head as I studied my new surroundings. Had these people gone through what I had gone through? Was it better for them or did they have it tougher than me? My first impression of the scene, or more specifically the men on the scene was they seemed to be promiscuous and predatory. There were bodies everywhere, good looking, fit guys; some where out of their heads on drink or drugs and others were just high on sexual tension. It was a place where I could have fun and let go while remaining sensible. Tim and I had loads of fun; most of the time was spent laughing. It was clear that he had the same feelings towards the same sex as I did, however I remember his time at school to be plain sailing; he was well liked by both girls and boys. All the while we had gone through school we never quite trusted each other enough to say how we felt about being gay. I know that I had suppressed my feelings so tightly down into the pit of my stomach that nothing would have shifted it. At this time I still didn't confess to Tim about my being gay and my relationship with Andrew.

After that first night on the scene I found I was going out onto the scene every Saturday night, it was like a drug. I could never consider myself to be a party animal; I had always had a good night at a pub but nightclubs... me? I found I didn't recognise myself as I used to. I had to go whether I wanted to or not. Preparation started early on those Saturday mornings, I was straight into Cardiff for a sun-bed at 8:00am after dropping Andrew at work, then home to clean the house and then the rest of the day was spent on body maintenance. By 6:00pm I was plucked, shaved, tanned and raring to go. I was off to my sanctuary where I was surrounded by tons of others who were all in the same boat as me, a place where I wouldn't be judged for being myself and where they played the best music. I didn't drink alcohol at all when I was on the scene, not being a very big drinker I found I had a better time on water, being naturally hyper I didn't need drugs either. I just run at my best when I am having a good time with good people.

There was something that should have received my utmost attention before my tanning, waxing and plucking ritual. That was **my** 'coming out' - well at least to those on the scene. In actual fact it might have been a good place to start. When people wanted to know more about me when I was out on the scene I told them I wasn't gay, it was something I was used to saying, therefore it felt easier and beside which Andrew and I were still hiding in the closet. Understandably there were those who didn't take kindly to me saying this especially when I submerged myself into their world and was obviously gay. This raised a lot of questions that needed resolving. I was going through a massive change in my life; it was like adolescence all over again. My body had changed but the transformation needed to happen inside.

I was learning about me and the world that existed outside the four walls of the home where I had been born. I had a craving inside to be in a relationship, well I was in a relationship, however Andrew and I were "just good friends" so everyone thought. I wanted to be public about our feelings for one another, I didn't want to walk through town holding hands or demonstrating other public displays of affection. Nevertheless I wanted the people who mattered to me to know that I was gay, and that Andrew was the person I was going to spend the rest of my days with, and not just a figment of my imagination. Andrew was not so keen on the idea, he was happy as we were, but I wasn't. It made it difficult when I went out to explain to people that I wasn't gay and I wasn't interested in them.

Needless to say it does nothing for one's self-esteem when you are in a relationship and you are unable to share it with others, how people who have affairs manage I will never know. My self-worth wasn't exactly running at peak levels when out on the scene. With my concealed feelings and my hidden relationship I held onto the virtues I had been born with. I wanted monogamy, however other people's promiscuous advances made me feel attractive and alive, and although I rejected them I knew something had to change.

Opening The Closet Door

It all came to a head one dark cold and wet evening in October 2003. After many heart to hearts with Denzil, who was gay and hugely popular at the call centre where we worked, I decided to come out. Denzil had experienced everything I was to take on. I met his mother a few weeks previously and she told me that my parents will still love me when I come out. This was a boost I really needed. After a tiring day at work I situated myself on the floor in front of the fire in the lounge. I called my parents, it was a "now or never" situation. I called Mam and Dad in South Africa, Mam answered and I told her I had something to tell her and I didn't think she would love me any longer. She replied "There is nothing you could say that would stop me from loving you". I didn't know what I was going to say, after that build up you can hardly go back. I couldn't even say the words "I am gay", every time I tried I choked, I physically choked. The only thing I could say was "Mam, I am like Denzil". Thankfully, I had told her about Denzil many times before; she knew he was a close friend and that he was gay. I spoke to my parents about him in the same way I did with all my other friends; they have always taken a keen interest in my friends. After this bombshell the line went quiet for a moment. I was mortified. Was silence good, or was it bad? I asked her to tell Dad and to call me back; she reassured me that he would be fine about it. Two minutes passed which felt like an eternity so I called them straight back. Those two minutes in gay terms felt like a lifetime when you have just admitted to your mother that you are just like Denzil! I am now in floods of tears, I was left wondering if I had lost everything or would my life be different to how I knew it. The first thing I said to Mam as she answered was "You didn't call me back"! Mam immediately asked "Do you want to speak to your Dad?" I replied, "No, I don't". The next voice on the phone was my Dad, "Hello matey" he said and then I knew everything was alright.

Dad and I have never had what some see as a normal father and son relationship, it was better! I very rarely call him Dad; we always use any words other than those titles that are commonly accepted in polite society. I call him Cheese, and he calls me Biscuits or Onions. It sounds really stupid when I am sat here typing it for all to see, but I am proud of our relationship. The terms do get more vulgar, I call him Arseholes and he will call me something equally as crude, just because it is funny. Well it is to us. No matter what happens to me in life, whether I am dealt a good hand or bad, I will always be allowed to smile because I have been given the gift of a wonderful childhood and wonderful parents. I can't remember the first time Dad told me he was proud of me because he has told me all too often. It is the love I receive from my parents that has helped me through turbulent times.

Coming out that evening was the hardest thing I have ever had to do. My parents were brilliant about my coming out and have been ever since. They accepted it right away, Mam was more shocked than Dad, he did say that he had an idea what was being said on that first phone call to Mam that evening. It is interesting how Dad knew; I could have been ringing to ask if I could borrow £20,000 or perhaps remortgage the house so I could buy the entire contents of Louis Vuitton, yet somehow he knew. He said "I have always known you were a bit light on your loafers" and Mam said "I would never have guessed". I found both responses highly amusing. Up to this point, I only outted myself, they knew nothing of Andrew, they didn't ask and I didn't tell them. I thought that it was best to let things take their own natural course. In time they learned about Andrew and from that day they have loved him just as they do my brother and sister-in-law.

I can appreciate it now, although I couldn't at the time, how draining it is re-adjusting to a new life. Old suppressed feelings and emotions had been released after years and years of containment, my shoulders felt lighter and there was a pleasant emptiness inside. This did take its toll on me mentally on the other hand. The mental strain that has been so draining for so long had gone, and with it states of depression washed over me like a tidal wave, it came with no warning and the effects were indescribable. First I couldn't control my emotions, I found myself crying over the silliest things, and my dreams were removed and replaced with nightmares. Each evening I went to bed only to dream of the death of yet another friend or family member, I was desperately unhappy, I lost over a stone in weight. I was eating properly, Andrew made sure of that. The weight just fell off me. Unbeknown to me at the time there were many of my loved ones worried about my rapid weight loss. Andrew, Auntie Joyce, my brother and sister in law were concerned, the news had even reached Mam and Dad in South Africa. They never expressed their concern to me; they called nearly everyday as normal and just listened when I needed to talk. I had reached a point where I looked terminally ill; I don't think my shaved head helped either. I went to the doctor and explained my symptoms, it was then it was diagnosed as depression. The first thing he wanted to do was prescribe anti-depressants, I refused the prescription because no matter how weak I was at the time, my mind had enough fight to say that I was going to overcome it without the aid of prescription drugs. It was an uphill struggle, each day it would be there waiting for me as I woke up and it was there until I closed my eyes at night: it was there if I woke in the night as the result of a bad dream. I was never away from it. With the power of positive thinking and a supportive and loving family it subsided. It went in the same way it had come, it just washed away. I suffered for nine months and for a long while I lived in fear of when it might return again. Thankfully it didn't and it won't. It was a process I needed to go through as I waved goodbye to the old me.

All The World's A Stage

They say that as one person enters the world another person leaves. William Shakespeare supposed that all the world is a stage, and all the men, women, yes even the gays are merely players. We have our exits and our entrances. In April 2004 our Nephew, William came into the world the day before his Uncle Andrew's Birthday. As someone who has always loved children and having dealt with the fact early on that I would never have children of my own, I remember the first time I held William and just being caught up in the emotion of realising that he was my little man and feeling that overwhelming instinct of protecting "your own".

Things were going swimmingly by this point, Andrew and I had bought our own home that was being built on the seafront in West Wales, Andrew's parents had bought a house there and we followed suit buying a house across the road.

In April 2005 we celebrated the 50th Birthday of Andrew's mother, Cheryl. It was a quiet celebration that consisted of special friends and family. We had a wonderful evening, we laughed, we ate and we made plans for the future like the trip to Florida that we had promised ourselves and put off. The evening came to an end. The following day, Friday, we paid a visit to his parents after work, Cheryl was not herself, we stayed a while and then went home for food. We often ate with them however we didn't on this particular evening. Andrew's Dad, Martin phoned later that evening and mentioned to Andrew that Cheryl was not feeling too well so Andrew asked for her to come to the phone. At the time she was watching some programme on Robbie Williams, she cut the call short saying "I've got to go, I've got to go". She was fine so we thought, and so she thought.

At around 3:00am on that Saturday morning, unbeknown to us an ambulance drove quietly into our little cul-de-sac to collect his mother. She had woken in the night and asked Martin to call an ambulance; she must have been unwell as she didn't like hospitals or ambulances. We received a call at around 5:30am for Andrew to go to hospital, he got ready and went. I couldn't sleep so I watched Mariah Carey being interviewed on David Letterman. Andrew then called me to go to the hospital. I asked if everything was alright and he said that everything was fine, I showered quickly and dressed and I was there in no time at all. I parked the car, as I walked across the car park I saw him coming towards me, his face said it all and as I got closer he mouthed the words "she died". I can't describe my feelings even now, not to mention how he was feeling. I wanted so much to take his pain away and at the same time I just wanted to run away. I wanted to drive until I reached the end of the earth by which time the pain surely would have gone. She had a massive heart attack and there was nothing they could have done for her, they fought to keep her alive, if she had lived she would have been brain damaged and she would not have wanted that. Her last words to him, when she said "I've got to go, I've got to go" I know for a fact these words remain with him today.

Time passed and the seasons came and went with most of the days feeling like a constant winter, one uneventful day replaced another. Uneventful was good, uneventful meant no additional pain or heartache; it meant we could get used to life as we knew it without Cheryl without any other gut wrenching alterations.

A New Direction

A year later I flew to South Africa to spend a few months with Mam and Dad, I arrived the day before Dad was due to have a second medical procedure on his back. His back was damaged in his youth, he worked in construction and one day picked a fight with a jack hammer and won... just! However, his victory did come at a price. His doctor told him soon after, he would be wheelchair bound by the time he was forty, thankfully this never happened but today he has limited strength in one leg and severe on-going back problems.

When he had made a full recovery I was on a plane heading back to South Wales, while I was away I made the decision to leave my role as a Customer Service Representative in the call centre. I knew that I needed to pursue my ambition of conquering the world of recruitment.

After four gruelling interviews with a recruitment agency that was based in the same office block as my Customer Services role, I secured myself a position in December 2006. That Christmas Mam and Dad returned home to South Wales for good. I began work in the January and was assigned to dealing with candidates in the field of architecture. My position was that of Recruitment Resourcer and it was my role to find the best architects and all manner of architectural candidates in the land. I started off a little jerky, but soon made the role my own, I was given no limitations, I took the role and just ran with it. I did whatever I liked and whatever I was doing, seemed to work. I knew for a fact that there were some reservations within the office of taking on "a gay". I very quickly dispelled any misgivings they might have had. I was a good friend to my colleagues and candidates alike. By this time, having come through so much in school and in my personal life, I was not going to give up what I wanted to do because people wondered whether they could get on with a gay, or if someone who is gay might or might not be good for business. I was myself and I won everyone over, I was popular within my office and in neighbouring offices and I was a big hit with both clients and candidates simply due to the fact I was myself and nothing else.

This was a time of change, a new job with better money, it was going well. I also found a new friend, Jay, who was not only a good friend but also a family member that I didn't really know before. I first noticed him working behind the bar when I began visiting the gay scene after returning from South Africa in 2002, he seemed familiar to me. I was convinced he was the absolute double of a young boy in a photograph hung on the wall of my great Auntie Doreen's home. He looked like the adult version of this little boy who was around six years old in the photograph. I had seen this photograph many times over the years but never met him. As soon as I saw him I was convinced it was him although I never said anything. Years passed and then I spotted him on FaceBook, it was then I knew that it was in fact him, and he was my cousin. Since then we have become close, in the same way our fathers were when they were growing up but drifted apart when they married. I often think how my life might have been easier having had Jay in my life growing up, he might have understood what I was going through and vice versa. It doesn't do any good dwelling on these circumstances and it's just a good job we have found one another but it does make me wonder.

Things became uneasy at work for me when the credit crunch of 2008 hit the world's economy. The architectural market began slowing which impacted upon my place of work profoundly with redundancies. Within time my colleagues were being affected by redundancies, month by month more and more vacant desks were appearing. The office that was once home to nearly twenty strong individuals, some of life's biggest characters began to dwindle too. The office seemed to grow bigger and bigger as the people got less and less. The banter and laughter that had once filled the air was knocking back and forth against the barren walls and sounded like a distant echo. You could look around the office and see the shadows of those who had one occupied the missing spaces. This does sound hugely sentimental however this was the mood of those I worked with.

A Happy New Year

By January 2009 the credit crunch had hit South Wales in the same way it did the rest of the world. It grew like a cancer that was out of control, jobs were scarce and candidates were flocking in their droves to find work in the architectural sector, a field that they had trained long and hard to work within. I required the energy I would use in a normal day's work just to get me out of bed. Each day was like fighting a losing battle; it became more difficult to recruit for architectural positions that did not exist.

On the 29th of April, Andrew and I settled in front of the television to celebrate our eight year anniversary together. I was awakened at 5:15am the following morning to the ringing of my mobile phone. I heard Dad's voice; I asked if everything was okay and he said "I need you to be a brave boy", I just froze and it was then he told me Auntie Joyce had passed away in the early hours of the morning. The phone fell from my hands; shocked, crying and in total disbelief I came crashing down not long after it. Andrew took the call and asked what had happened; I could hear Dad start to explain so I ran and headed for the spare bedroom. I didn't want to know, so I scrambled away, I was in a blind panic. I couldn't speak, it was as if someone had gripped me by the throat, I got back into bed, and was instantly transported back to the six days previous when I saw her for the last time. When everything was going so well, reality had to bite. I showered, did my hair, got dressed and went to work. I shouldn't have gone, I still couldn't speak. I didn't stay there long, I couldn't.

She died at the age of seventy-six years old, from an aneurism; she went the same way as Nanny Beatrice, who also died at the same age, and to me it was as if history was repeating itself.

The funeral took place in the same church where we held Nanny's funeral twenty years previously. It was as if no time had passed at all, so many things had happened in the twenty years, these were forgotten as it felt like nothing else had happened. The one difference was I was twenty years older, so I was old enough to be pall bearer this time. I held her coffin so tightly and buried my head into the side of it. I didn't want to let her go. At every stage of my life Auntie Joyce had always been there fighting my corner. She was so many things to me as well as my bingo buddy. She was the biggest character that ever blessed the earth and I was very lucky to have had her.

Two weeks came and went and then I was made redundant from the job I was so good at. The role I executed with pride and passion was taken away because of the dire state of the global economic climate. I was sad to be leaving the friends I had made, but I knew that I was put on this planet for a greater purpose other than to line the pockets of higher executives. I was destined to make a difference to people's lives, to make their world a better place and to help those who wanted to get the best experiences from life so I started on the path of Life Coaching.

The Birth of True Colours Coaching

Going through life and experiencing periods of change is inevitable and for many it is uncomfortable and I am usually one of those, however, I embraced my redundancy. I was not a bit sorry for being superfluous to the requirements of my former employer; I received the wake up call that had perhaps been long overdue. Andrew and I went out that evening with the family to celebrate my redundancy; we went to our favourite Chinese restaurant. It was that day I decided that I was never going to feel the feelings of being "redundant" again. I decided to go it alone, start my own successful business and help others to get all that they want from life; this was the birth of *True Colours Coaching*.

True Colours Coaching was born from one of my most positive experiences and that was redundancy. My position as Life Coach is one that comes with more responsibility than I imagined possible, conversely it is a position that allows me to spring out of bed each morning because I get to assist amazing and wonderful people both gay and straight to get to grips with life and create a world that is right for them. I can appreciate what it is like to get up each and everyday in a world where you feel like an outsider looking in or where you question your place in this big wide world. When you feel that you were born different to the rest of the world, it undeniably takes its toll on every part of your emotional, mental and physical energy. You will one day realise that you will celebrate your uniqueness, whatever that difference may be.

Your uniqueness will make you stand out and shine from those that brush past you on the street or sit opposite you on the commuting journey to work. You were born different for a purpose, not so that you can feel isolated and aloof from the rest, but so you have a different story to tell. Taking the first step can seem a daunting task, however once you have started with that one step; the remaining journey will become easier. It can be difficult to motivate yourself to get out of bed in the morning to get to school, to work or back into the workplace having had some time away. There is no need to be unhappy in school or work, you tailor your life so it suits you rather than being conditioned to work as others see fit. You are more powerful than you credit yourself.

There is a reason you have stumbled across this book or across me. If you feel that you need to drop me an email or give me a call then please do so. The experience of Life Coaching will equip you with the tools you require to live the life that you want. You need to decide when you truly want to take the first step to a brighter, happier you.

I am very proud of what I have achieved and I am proud of the business that I have created. It wasn't created by me alone; it was born from the continued help, love and support of my friends and family. *True Colours Coaching* has helped and is currently helping so many talented individuals discover who they are and to live the life they want. If you believe, you can achieve!

The Law Of Attraction - And So The Lesson Begins

If I were to conclude with a summary of the events that shaped my life, I would have to say this. I was born lucky with the wonderful gifts with which I was bestowed. I have a family which I am proud of, I have met some wonderful people and continue to do so and I am continuously making new friends. I have learned that there are those who you will not or cannot get along with, however if you avoid them and they avoid you it makes for a happy existence on both sides. My parents always advised me to treat people as I would like to be treated. I find it difficult to do this, probably because it is something that relates to me, so I just treat people in the same way I would like a member of my family to be treated.

I am now a firm believer that my life has been mapped out for me and that the mind creates what it manifests. It is called the *Law of Attraction*. Some people believe that babies choose their parents before they are born – I can't quite see that somehow but it's a nice thought, if not a bit odd. The Law of Attraction has brought so many wonderful people into my life and they came at I time when I needed them. I didn't know what they would look like but I somehow knew I needed them and they needed me. It happened the day I met Andrew on the staircase at his Nan's home. It happened when I met Rhiannon, we became best friends at school during our GCSE years - she wanted to chop my bits off during a woodwork class when we met because I jokingly said she fancied someone who she did not like – it wasn't the best ice-breaker. Had I not been a quick thinker I could have easily become a eunuch. Wendy came into my life just when I needed her, it was just after my depression, and we became instant friends and have been close ever since. I met my friend Angelina whilst working in Recruitment, she was the Trainer but I had seen her many times before in the elevator whilst I was working for another employer in my Customer Services role (both companies were in the same building). She was always smartly dressed and wore the most amazing stilettos – fabulous! For many years I knew her only as the girl with amazing shoes but when I changed companies she then became a best friend. The Law of Attraction also has a way of playing tricks too. I met Lynsey, my

Colonic Hydrotherapist when I attended my first session. Colonic irrigation was something I always wanted to try before I died. I walked into the private clinic where she worked to find that it was Lynsey who was in the same year as me in Comprehensive School. We hardly said two words to each other in school, we smiled and greeted one another when we walked around the school yard and that was that. Now Lynsey is a trusted friend who has seen bits of me that very few people have seen. Each of my friends come with a story, I will not bore you with them all but if you want only good people in your life then focus on their attributes and those people will find you. You do however need to go out and try and find them too. Again this is the same way I met my cousin Jay – granted it did happen a bit late in life, but better to happen late than not happen at all.

I often thought that my life has been one big coincidence and many times wondered if it was all part of an elaborate plot. The series of events that have played through my life have happened at a specific point for a reason. If I had done things differently I might not be here now, I might be somewhere else. I could be happier if I had changed things, although I very much doubt it. I have always wanted to write this book, I mapped it out once and then threw it away. I then decided to pursue it when my employer said they no longer required my services, just because one person didn't require my services I knew that there were many who did and this book has now been printed to do that.

I finish by wishing you luck in everything you do. The most important things of all; just be yourself, make the decisions that you feel are right for you, focus upon and imagine what it is you want and with time it will happen. As you look back you will then see that what you have achieved is not too dissimilar to what you imagined to be possible.

About True Colours Coaching

At True Colours Coaching we endeavour to deliver a rewarding coaching experience through maintaining our integrity, being devoted to our client's goals and allowing them to express their individuality and enjoy the life they deserve.

Our mission is to provide a personalised coaching service that empowers, each and every client to excel to greatness through positive exploration and celebrate their individuality with good humour, lots of laughter and plenty of smiles.

"If you always do what you have always done, you will always get what you've always got". So why make do with what you have, try something new and who knows where you will be if you decide to make those changes you have been putting off.

True Colours Coaching can assist in making a more rewarding life in the areas of:

Heath ▪ Wealth/ Finances ▪ Relationship ▪ Being Different ▪ Spiritual ▪ Personal Fulfilment ▪ Career Change / Progression ▪ Family Circumstances ▪ Motivation ▪ Confidence ▪ Self-esteem

Or anything else that you feel need improvement and helps to get out of bed each morning with a smile on your face and a spring in your step.

"What is life coaching?" I hear you ask. Well, it is a partnership between you and me which requires passion, dedication and 100 per cent commitment from both parties. My role as a Life Coach is to assist the client, that's you, every step of the way to define and clarify your dreams and goals to ensure that they are fulfilled in a timely fashion. You will expect to both see and enjoy the success that you deserve and I will expect results, results and results. I will work with you only when you guarantee that you are 100 per cent committed to getting the life you want.

He also works with businesses of all size, large and small to help them get the most out of what they have, and explore new opportunities. But, unlike others Richard sees the business world as people centred. Without the important cogs the machine just won't function. People need nourishing and encouraging to get the best of their untapped ability.

www.TrueColoursCoaching.com

About The Author

Richard is a Life Coach who applies life coaching holistically to those who feel different to the rest of the world, for whatever reason, not just because of their sexuality.

"We are imperfect people living in an imperfect world, yet we get singled out for not being perfect. "

Richard Harris

Richard benefited from attending one of the toughest 'Schools of Life' from the age of three, and he remained there until he was eighteen. He then took a little time out to live in Canada and then returned to join the rat run. He worked within the corporate field of car insurance spanning customer service, sales and training and then moved into the rollercoaster world of recruitment dealing with candidate generation, candidate development, client liaison and in-house training specialising in the disciplines of Architecture and Social Housing.

True Colours Coaching was born after Richard experienced one of life's most positive and life changing experiences, redundancy. He made the decision that no-one was ever going to make his position redundant again and discovered that he was actually invincible.

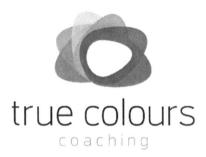

true colours
coaching

DISCOUNT VOUCHER

As a Thank You for investing your precious time, effort, and money into enjoying Closets Are For Clothes, I would like to extend my gratitude by giving you a discount on my Life Coaching and Hypnotherapy service.

If you wish to take up this offer then please visit the True Colours Coaching website at **www.TrueColoursCoaching.com** and get in touch, mention the book and discount code **CAFCTY**.

INDEX OF CASE STUDIES

Lightning Source UK Ltd.
Milton Keynes UK
21 May 2010

154477UK00003B/7/P